THE HEALING MIND

THE HEALING MIND

You Can Cure Yourself Without Drugs

by

DR. IRVING OYLE
Director, Bolinas Headlands Healing Service

Foreword by Stanley Krippner, Ph.D.
President, Association for Humanistic Psychology

CELESTIAL ARTS
Millbrae, California

Also by Dr. Oyle:
Magic, Mysticism, and Modern Medicine

First Printing, June 1975
Made in the United States of America

Library of Congress Cataloging in Publication Data

Oyle, Irving, 1925—
    The healing mind.

    1. Therapeutics, Suggestive. 2. Mind and body.
3. Medicine and psychology. I. Title.
RC498.Q94   615'.851   74-10069
ISBN: 0-912310-80-4

FOREWORD

Irving Oyle organized New York City's first free clinic. While some young people were engulfed in the raptures of LSD and the worlds which it revealed, others were suffering from bad trips, frightening visions, and blown minds. It was these casualties of the psychedelic age who showed up at Oyle's clinic to be made whole again and to "get it all together."

The Spencer Memorial Presbyterian Church, of which I was an officer, supported much of Oyle's work. And it was at Spencer Church that Oyle and I first served on a panel which discussed the role of psychedelic experience in religion. We appeared in public several times, supporting a holistic approach to medicine, an experiential approach to religion, and a close look at the country's marijuana laws. As far back as 1967, we had advocated the decriminalization approach to marijuana eventually adopted by the presidential commission in 1972. Oyle and I even appeared before the New York State legislative advisory subcommittee and at a breakfast for legislators in Albany, New York, urged lower marijuana penalties. The plan we proposed was adopted by the State of Oregon in 1973 and, in a 1974 evaluation, Oregon's district attorneys reported no discernible increase in marijuana usage.

Oyle and I realized that, like any drug, marijuana had the potential for abuse, especially if used constantly and in large amounts. However, we felt that the invasion of one's personal privacy had a far greater capacity for abuse, especially when one considered the thousands of individuals in prison for possession of small portions of marijuana.

When Oyle moved to California, it was again a Presbyterian church that supported his clinic. I invited him to Novato to meet Mickey Hart, a musician friend of mine who had set up a recording studio on his ranch. Another visitor at Hart's ranch was Rolling Thunder, a Shoshone medicine man. Hart and I brought the shaman and the osteopath together with some trepidation, as this was Rolling Thunder's first serious encounter with a physician.

After several hours in the recording studio, they walked through the door, arm in arm. Oyle reported, "We compared our practices. Rolling Thunder said that when a patient comes to him, he makes a diagnosis, goes through a ritual, and gives the patient some medicine that will restore health. I replied that when a patient comes to me, I make a diagnosis and go through the ritual of writing a prescription which will give the patient some medicine to restore health. In both cases, a great deal of magic is involved—the type of magic called 'faith in one's doctor.'"

Rolling Thunder later agreed to join me as a member of the advisory board of Oyle's clinic in Bolinas. His knowledge of herbal medicine complemented Oyle's practice of osteopathy, traditional medicine, psychic healing, and Do-In (acupuncture massage).

During my several visits to Oyle's clinic, I was pleased to see the emphasis placed on the psychological etiology of the sickness. Patients were asked, "Why did you allow yourself to become ill?" These queries were in keeping with the philosophy of Rolling Thunder and other shamen I have known that most physical illness reflects a spiritual malaise; one must change one's way of life to remain healthy.

In 1972, Oyle had a chance to bring the attention of an international audience to his work in Bolinas. He was an invited speaker at the International Meeting on the Problems of Biological Energy held in Moscow. Sixty scientists from ten countries participated in the conference and Oyle described his utilization of evoked visual imagery to assist group healing effects on a patient.

In the Soviet Union, he heard a great deal about biological plasma, a hypothesized "fifth state of matter." Biological plasma is thought to be the medium through which telepathy, psychokinesis, and psychic healing takes place. It may penetrate an organism's physical body and it could even exist in such abundance as to form a "bioplasmic body." If so, such a phenomenon would have to affect the practice of medicine; it could be that attempts to restore the "bioplasmic body" to health would be simpler than work on the physical body—and may in turn bring about physical changes.

Irving Oyle is in touch with the new developments in healing throughout the world. Unlike many physicians who speculate and dabble in the unorthodox while conducting their medical practices in the same old way, Oyle puts his new knowledge directly to use. I hope that this book will spread the word of his type of medicine to more people and even persuade a few physicians to give some of Oyle's procedures a try. Both the physician and the patient are due to benefit if holistic medicine begins to catch on in offices and clinics around the world.

Stanley Krippner, Ph.D.
President, Association for Humanistic Psychology

THE HEALING MIND

I

"You gotta give me something to stop this pain or I'm gonna kill myself!"

He walked rapidly around the room making deep raspy moaning sounds. He was unable to open his mouth because of swelling and spasm of the jaw muscles. On further examination and what little information came from his immovable mouth, it was determined that a molar, probably rotten and abscessed, was giving him unbearable pain. No narcotics are stored in the clinic and the dentist was out fishing. The only resort was a therapy untried and unknown. I had earlier decided that the next 30–40 patients who came into the clinic would be treated with sonopuncture, and here was my first case!

Sonopuncture was derived from my clinical interest in acupuncture wedded to a well-practiced reliance on ultrasound therapy. I selected an acupuncture point on the back of the hand that is used to produce sufficient analgesia to permit thyroidectomy operations in China. The ultrasound was applied through a quartz crystal on a layer of mineral oil; the vibrating head placed against the appropriate acupuncture point. (In standard ultrasound treatments, the head is placed directly over the site of pain or spasm.) Ultrasound, directed through the vibrating crystal, is a well-established safe, and painless procedure, and avoids the stress of submitting to the traditional needle method.

The sonopuncture treatment continued for about ten minutes and within five minutes after completion the patient fell asleep. When he awoke 30 minutes later he had some discomfort but the acute emergency had subsided. Two days later he returned, still not having seen a dentist, and informed me that the pain and swelling had gone: "If it don't bother me, I don't bother it."

The sonopuncture treatment was continued on the next 32 patients arriving at the clinic. The type of ailment treated was typical of those treated by any family physician: anxiety, depression, localized pain (back, shoulder, elbow), poison oak, burns, bruises, painful menstrual periods. Each patient demonstrated marked clinical improvement within 24 hours, some within 30 minutes after treatment. Abscesses opened, burns healed, rashes disappeared before our eyes—we were getting excellent therapeutic responses in 70% of a random sample of general practice complaints. In addition, there seemed to be a marked tranquilizing or sedative effect, sometimes lasting for several days. Five patients noted increased clarity of vision and intensified color perception. [1]

The clinic, Headlands Healing Service, is located in Bolinas, a small coastal town north of San Francisco. It opened its doors in 1970, looking for ways to improve medical care. The clinic operates independently of other clinics and hospitals, and is dedicated to consideration and development of cures that do not rely on chemotherapy or surgery.

This current California experiment serves a population with great diversity. Some people live in tree houses while others come to spend time in expensive vacation homes. The area is an excellent cross section of the whole country in terms of income, age, etc. My initial practice was in a suburban community near New York City with subsequent practices in the Lower East Side of Manhattan and among the native Indians of Mexico. All locations were essential steps in my evolution from a family physician to a humanitarian teacher.

When I graduated from the Philadelphia College of Osteopathic Medicine and Surgery in 1953, I was aware of the fact that there were some ten drugs in the pharmacopoeia which served all the needs of a general medical practitioner. You could do it all with those ten drugs. I bought a little black bag, filled it with the ten drugs, went out and did it. What I was *doing* was healing: sick people came to me. By using a combination of these ten basic drugs, I helped them get well.

As time went on, this began to change—healing became more difficult. In the course of general practice, there are always the inevitable, fatal cancer cases, the sudden heart attacks, kidney disease, and the like. I learned that my ten trusty drugs were not omnipotent; there was no combination that could offer some patients even a glimmer of hope. At this point the physician usually says, helplessly, "There is nothing more that can be done." The patient with a terminal disease is advised to go home and finish the affairs of living. If necessary, a hospital bed can be arranged.

Despite my realization that the ten drugs did not include a panacea, I continued to accept an occasional failure philosophically. During my internship, I considered myself a whiz-bang at treating heart failure. I was convinced that I understood the pathophysiology. This confidence was translated into therapeutic success on may occasions. One day a patient was admited to my service with early congestive heart failure.

"Fear not," I told him, "we'll have you back home in no time at all."

After listening patiently to the scenario of how one drug would drain the excess fluid from his bloodstream while another increased the tone and contractile power of his heart muscle, and yet a third would dissolve all his anxieties and worries, he said quietly, "Forget it, Doc, I'm ready to move on."

"Don't be silly," I retorted, "I never miss when I treat heart failure."

But I missed! Three days after admission, in spite of all our efforts, his heart stopped beating.

This case raises these questions: Did the patient make it

stop by an act of his will? Why didn't a highly effective treatment plan work in this case? Does the patient's *will to live*
affect the outcome? How?

Sometime after this incident a staff conference was held in
the hospital and this case was presented. No answers were
forthcoming regarding these questions. The patient had been
signed out with a final diagnosis of *arteriosclerotic heart
disease with congestive heart failure.* We agreed on a diagnosis
which explains nothing. We simply employed scientific
semantics to label medical failure. We didn't know why a
treatment which worked for most patients, failed for this one.
We didn't know if a patient could stop his heart and end his
own life by an act of will. We didn't want to believe our
medicines, effective in most cases, could not overcome the
patient having lost the *will to live.* Only recently have we
begun to understand more about the psychological and
physical causes of heart attacks and, as a result, gain insight
into the relationship between mental attitude and disease. [2]

People most likely to die of heart attacks are those who
worry a great deal about their social responsibilities. They
tend to be conscientious workers whose lives are run on a tight
time schedule, referred to by doctors as Type A. Type A people
tend to be compulsive empiricists, exhibiting what Jung called
a *cramp of consciousness.* This attitude is represented in the
body by a physiologic state which Hans Selye, a prominent
research physiologist, calls the alarm state. [3]

Selye recently reassessed his earlier findings and con-
cluded that this state can give rise to different, usually chronic,
ailments in different individuals. He has further determined
that "conditioning factors" serve to either avoid manifestation
or enhance the effect of stress. These factors may have been
arrived at through the parents, the age of the individual, the
sex, or many other external conditioning factors. Also, they
have been arrived at by internal conditioning such as chemotherapy or diet. Subjected to one or more of these factors, an
otherwise tolerated "degree of stress can become pathogenic
and cause diseases of adaptation which affect predisposed
areas of the body selectively." [4] If you worry a lot it doesn't take
much to make you seriously ill; the diseases of stress are hang-

ing over our heads awaiting the agent that will cut them free to crash into our lives.

For animals, including modern man, this normal *fight or flight* reaction to stress is essential for survival. The blood supply of the body is shunted from the areas near the skin to the muscles and to vessels deep in the body. This minimizes the blood loss in case of violation of the skin line of defense. Violent hormonal changes occur which raise the blood pressure, increase heart rate, and shift total bodily energies from maintenance to defense systems. The entire organism is placed on *red alert*, prepared to battle for its life or flee from imminent danger.

For example, a jungle-dwelling man might go into the alarm state when confronted by a hungry tiger. The reaction is mediated by the adrenal cortical hormones, one of which is adrenaline. Within several minutes or an hour, a day on the outside, either the man is dead or the tiger is dead or the man has escaped to safety. But suppose the precipitating stressor is not a tiger. Suppose it is your boss at the office, your wife or husband at home, or the teacher at school. Type A people exhibit this mobilized state in a traffic tie-up if they happen to be late for an appointment or in a hurry to get home. As they go from one stressful situation to another, the hormonal alarm system reacts as if the cause were actually a hungry tiger threatening life itself. Type A Homo sapiens live in a state of chronic alarm. Blood vessels are constantly contracted, the heart beats with increased force and at an accelerated rate against resistant blood vessels, palms are constantly sweaty, breathing is shallow and restricted. The brain's dominant hemisphere broods and keeps alive stressful situations of the past and tries to wrestle with an imaginary future. There is usually no violent physical release for this mobilized and pent-up energy. Prolonging this uptight state causes the parts of the body to wear out.

There is a group of afflictions called *disease of stress*. Arteriosclerosis (hardening of the arteries), and many forms of arthritis and heart disease fall into this category. How prevalent are these diseases? How often are they the cause of death? "The great change in the nature of the health problem during this century is illustrated by a comparison of the 10 leading causes of death in 1900 and in 1970. In 1900 three of the 10 (tuberculosis, influenza-pneumonia and diphtheria) were directly infectious and three more (gastroenteritis, chronic nephritis and diseases of early infancy) were closely related to the infectious processes. By 1970 none of the first 10 causes of death was an infectious disease except for influenza-pneumonia and certain diseases of early infancy, and in both of these groups the mortality rate was far below the level of 1900. Today the list is headed by heart disease, cancer and cerebro-vascular lesions—all chronic diseases. The first two have increased in terms of death per 100,000 people by 268 percent and 240 percent respectively since 1900. Other chronic diseases, such as general arteriosclerosis and diabetes, have emerged as leading causes of death. Of every 100 males born in the United States this year, 83 are likely to die eventually of a chronic disease; in 1901 the rate was 52 in 100. The likelihood of dying of an infectious disease is now about six in 100, which is about one-sixth of the rate in 1901."[5] For many victims caught in the vicious cycle of stress, worry, and increased stress, death is the only way out of an impossible situation. Many patients displaying physical symptoms of illness, have admitted to me, "My life is so screwed up, I'd be better off dead."

There are people who can leave the day's worries at the office, they know how to relax. Type B people allow themselves lapses of daydreaming and are able to periodically shut off empirical reality. They are less prone to fatal heart seizures. Most of them would subscribe to the old idea of the power of positive thinking. There are many groups who use this philosophy in teaching their followers that if they constantly see their situations in the most positive light, everything will be fine. "If you want to have lots of money," they say, "act as if you already have it. *See yourself spending it!* Assume that you have it and it will come to you." The same formula is applied to the goals of happiness, health and success.

Sir William Osler, a well-known Canadian medical authority, once said, "It is more important to know the patient than to know the disease." He further observed that our pathologists are regaling us with detailed descriptions of new pathological conditions. He wondered whether they might be creating these new diseases by their vivid descriptions. This is often referred to as iatrogenic or "doctor caused" disease.

The oath of Hippocrates requires that I administer no poisons to my patients even if I am requested to do so. The ancient teacher also advised his students that the first law of healing was, "Above all, don't make things worse." In a report from the World Health Organization, we are advised that one of every four people who die in hospitals is killed by drugs. It is believed that this is because physicians are unfamiliar with the dangers of new drugs which they freely prescribe. The same report informs us that 70% of the drugs now in use were not being prescribed when half of today's physicians were in medical school. [6]

The drug companies, in a recent Senate hearing, did not challenge estimates that the misuse of drugs kills 30,000 people annually, and that 50,000 to 100,000 additional patients die from treatment-resistant bacteria which have emerged in part because of misuse and overuse of antibiotics. [7]

At the same hearing, Senator Edward Kennedy (Democrat, Massachusetts) claimed "that physicians are inadequately educated about drugs in medical school, become confused by the use of 20,000 brand names for 700 drug entities, and being busy, tend to rely excessively for drug information on manufacturers."

In spite of these alarming statistics, drug use by physicians continues to escalate. A team of infectious disease specialists from the University of Wisconsin notes, "We are now in an era of explosion in the use of all drugs." A prominent American internist, Charles E. Mengel, University of Missouri, observes, "...significant amounts of disease are, in fact, produced by apparently therapeutic maneuvers." He feels that the responsibility lies with the advertising media, the pharmaceutical industry, and the lay population. The infectious disease specialists agree: "...it is quixotic to blame physicians for the overuse of drugs, when their patients and the nature of medical practice demand that they provide something for an unending series of complaints." [8]

The physician who forgets his oath to *administer no poisons* must bear prime responsibility, and forego the luxury of blaming patients, advertisers, or anyone else.

When all things are considered, the war against humanity's ancient enemy, infectious disease, is going badly for our side. Faithful above all to the law of cause and effect, the medical researchers applied Koch's postulates from bacteriology and gained some spectacular victories. Smallpox has been eliminated from the Western hemisphere, polio and tuberculosis have been beaten back, to name just three. However, in the area of infections of the kidney and bladder, the tide seems to be turning against us.

A recent drug company ad tells us that at any one time an estimated 8 million Americans have urinary tract infections. Over 20 million Americans have gonorrhea, many more have cancer, or one of a host of other *incurable* diseases. The organisms which we are told are responsible for urinary tract infection are no longer destroyed by our powerful, expensive antibiotics. In spite of this, each year the drugs become more powerful, costlier, and more dangerous. The simplistic "A pill for every ill" approach to disease has backfired. We are beginning to kill as many people with the cure as does the unchecked disease.

In 1968, I left Farmingdale and set up an experimental clinic on New York's Lower East Side. I thought I could get closer to the reality of a ritual necessary for universal healing. The neighborhood of East 10th Street and Avenue B was indeed closer and certainly real, but not quite what I had in mind. The clinic was sponsored by the Spencer Presbyterian Church in Brooklyn. The pastor, Reverend Glenesk, was anxious that his religion be relevant to the problems of humanity. Our purpose was to start a high-quality health care service in an urban ghetto area. The state of public health in this Lower East Side community was better than that among the Tarahumara, but inferior to that of the Mayas.

After two years on the Lower East Side, social conditions made it obvious that battlefield medicine was the major need of this area as it deteriorated and began engaging in active revolution. The experiment was discontinued and moved to the present rural area in California. The New York experiment had shown that it was possible to practice high-quality medicine even in the slums, provided the physician is really willing to do it. For that period, we had made it possible to consult with the best medical specialists—welfare patients were covered by health insurance which paid for consultations in fancy uptown office. Our consultants were usually heads of departments in local universities. Their social and financial positions were secure and they were glad to perform a service. As an extra inducement the city paid $25 per visit for seeing patients whom they would otherwise see free in the clinics. The medical standards of these specialists in their private offices was the same for all patients.

The ten basic drugs by now had expanded to a list of thousands. Phenobarbital had been replaced by a list of dozens of highly touted tranquilizers, none of which is more effective than properly administered barbiturates. These substitutes can be dangerous, and are far more costly. For example, in 1953, a single type of penicillin was effective in treating strep throat, pneumonia, abscesses, etc. Today, we have available at least 15 different types, all of which are very expensive and of limited value against increasingly resistant organisms. In our experiment on the Lower East Side, all the patients were on welfare and the emphasis was on prescribing the cheapest drug which was therapeutically effective. We were successful.

In my private practice, I had faced a problem of escalating curative doses. As time went on, I found myself prescribing larger and larger doses or moving to drugs with greater potency. If one of my patients came home from a business trip with a case of gonorrhea, I could give him 300,000 units of crystalline penicillin in a single shot for prophylaxis or for cure. The treatment solved the problem simply and efficiently. Not too many years later, county health officials were suggesting that maybe the dose should be doubled as the old treatment was no longer effective. As more resistant strains developed the recommended dosage increased to 1.2 million and finally went to 2.4 million units. Today gonorrhea, like inflation, continues to rage out of control. The treatment taught me at medical school was no longer working rapidly and consistently.

At any rate, many doctors today still insist that our best hope lies in more efficient weapons systems (stronger tranquilizers, antidepressants, antibiotics, etc.) administered in larger and larger doses. A young intern recently admitted to me, "In many fields, especially internal medicine, there is a definite need for improvement...in rheumatoid arthritis and the like, we dump in cortisone and we don't even know why; but you must admit that antibiotic therapy is the one great advance of Western medicine." I can admit that, yet it is alarming to note the rate at which drugs become obsolete and ineffective, and some drugs can cause serious illness—even death.

The one great source of healing energy utilized less and less as the medical arsenal escalates is the vital factor of the doctor-patient relationship. I learned early in practice that two elements had to be present in order for me to be an effective physician. First, I had to be convinced from my own experience that my reality structure and its healing system were valid and effective. I made a mental image which I tried to convey convincingly to the patient. For example, in a case of pneumonia, I would give the patient penicillin and create an image of the destructive organisms in the lung absorbing the antibiotic. This absorption caused them to swell and explode destroying themselves. Their extermination was manifested by the patient getting well—it was not even necessary for him to understand my model. If the patient believes that I know what I am doing and I firmly believe in my therapeutic ritual, healing usually takes place. On the other hand, as already discussed, if a patient chooses not to recover from an illness, there is very little that can be done to alter the course.

The autoimmune diseases are a group in which the body's own defense mechanism—antibodies—turns on itself as if carrying out a self-destruct program. Is the body in these cases responding to an unwitting command? Are diseases like rheumatoid arthritis and multiple sclerosis a subtle form of suicide? Does the patient's mental picture of the disease affect the course of that disease?

I am suggesting the possibility that we humans may regain control over the behavior of our own bodies. Physicians throughout history, such as the 16th century alchemist and physician, Paracelsus, and the 20th century contemporary of Freud, Carl Jung, have been attracted to the study of mental imagery as the quintessence of all healing rituals. The alchemists who founded modern medical practice, as well as the science of chemistry, taught that the panacea, the cure for all the ills of mankind, was to be created by means of the mystical marriage of the opposites. This can be done only by accepting the ability of the mind to control the matter making up the body. We breathe, our heart beats, we react to stop signs without conscious thinking, we grow our hair, and do so much more that we are not really aware of without conscious control. Could we reach the internal mechanism that triggers and maintains these processes, we could conceivably improve the health of many people.

II

In 1966, I was enjoying my life as a general practitioner in Farmingdale, New York, when I was presented with the opportunity to spend a short time in Mexico. The project, sponsored by the Jesuit mission involved several volunteer physicians in improving health conditions among the Indians of Sisoguichi in the Sierra Madre mountains of Chihuahua. It would be difficult to create a greater change of environment for a medical practice than from the middle-class Long Island community to the remote mountains of Mexico, where the patient load consisted mostly of cave-dwelling Tarahumara Indians. Instead of house calls, we made cave calls. This was man in his natural habitat, creating life for himself under the most primitive conditions.

The healing science of Western medicine was being transported to Cro-Magnon man. Life among these people had not changed in thousands of years. While many of the Indians died young from a variety of causes, the survivors lived to remarkable ages. A Jesuit padre flew us to a village located at an elevation of 10,000 feet in response to a radio message from the local priest. There we treated a man of indeterminate age and were directed by an 88-year-old lady to her mother's home.

Her mother had suffered from heart failure and was being maintained on digitalis. More important, the village matriarch, 107 years old, was interested in seeing the new "gringo" doctor.

Another trait besides longevity which was demonstrated by these primitive people was that of physical stamina. A common sport among the younger Tarahumara is the game of *bola*. This is a race which lasts as long as two days and nights, covering enormous distances. The families of the contestants run alongside carrying food and water. At night these helpers carry torches through the forest to keep visible the wooden ball which must be kicked from the starting line to the finish point. In another instance, a father walked 40 miles daily for a week to visit his six-year-old son in the mission hospital and to get home in time to give the evening penicillin dose to his wife and four other children—all of whom had pneumonia.

It was apparent that the subjective living experience of these people (how they felt from the time they awoke in the morning to the time they retired for the night) was very different from what I had seen in Farmingdale! It seemed that 35,000 years of evolution had done very little to change their subjective life experience.

The Indians also supplied an insight into healing, one which I did not understand at all. But there were areas in which it was extremely effective as demonstrated the following year during a similar work period with the Mayas in Yucatan. These people lived in a more advanced state of civilization than did the Tarahumara but depended on native healing rituals as did the Indians of central Mexico. In Chomula, I met a Mexican doctor in a small government clinic. When I asked to see his medical equipment, he smiled and showed me a modern treatment room which was in an advanced state of neglect. Some of the equipment showed signs of rust, "There is no need to maintain the stuff I never use. The Indian people do not use my services, they hardly recognize the existence of the Mexican government. They don't need me because their own medicine men are more effective healers, their methods get better results. I can't do for them what they can."

Here was a group of humans who, given a free choice between 20th century medicine and ancient Mayan medicine, chose the latter. The doctor was a Western-trained physician who had learned both systems firsthand, and made the same choice. "We work things out," he said. "The medicine man will sometimes add penicillin powder to his potions. I can't honestly say that it makes any difference in their therapeutic efficacy."

My confidence in my therapeutic system had already been shaken by my own observations and that conversation moved me along another notch.

The comparison of these two healing systems and their effectiveness can be enlightening. If you consult a modern American physician for a complaint, he performs a ritual which consists of X-rays, blood tests, and physical examination with medical tools. When he is finished he may say, for example, "You have an ulcer." He then proceeds to describe in detail an ulcerated area in the lining of your stomach which, being constantly bathed in hydrocloric acid, is prevented from healing. He may even explain with pictures or three-dimensional models how the process can eat into a blood vessel and cause bleeding or penetrate the wall to cause perforation—a catastrophe requiring immediate surgical intervention.

Having made the diagnosis and given the process a name, the physician recommends a program based on established practice. Even if it fails and the patient gets worse or dies, he is usually satisfied that he has earned his fee and discharged his responsibility to his patient. The patient, on the other hand, does not really know what initiated the chain of events, or how to alter their compelling course. Having a clear picture of impending disaster, he worries about it, thus stimulating its materialization.

I had been taught in medical school (and had practiced as a physician) that all I could do is create the conditions under which healing can take place. The Indian medicine man sees himself as a *channel* for cosmic healing energy. After all, the body is a self-repairing mechanism—it *has* the power to heal itself. Apparently some kind of ritual is necessary. Medicine men transmit religious or magical powers through ritual while the modern physician initiates healing through a rather formalized examination, diagnosis, and therapy. Even so, in either case, the dominant hemisphere of the brain receives information, processes it, and accepts or rejects the ritual as the truth. Some patients decide that only the proper herb can heal while others put childlike faith in the power of the pill; still others insist that salvation can be achieved by mastering a particular yoga position or by repeating a mantra. *Whatever you put your trust in can be the precipitating agent for your cure.* Recently, Dr. William Kroger made the following prediction: "...arthritics, then the asthmatics, the neurotics, and then the cancerous... Help will seem imminent to these—they will journey off to the Lourdes of acupuncture and throw down their crutches and their canes, not realizing that it's not the rock that cures, but their own inner belief." Any ritual accepted by the patient as reality can be substituted for the word *acupuncture.*

So it is possible that this inner belief is the vital factor in any healing process regardless of the ritual employed by the therapist healer. In the course of twenty years of family medical practice I became aware of two factors which are essential to the therapeutic relationship: the physician must have the complete confidence in his healing sytem or ritual, and the patient must trust that the physician knows what he is doing. If either aspect of this inner belief is missing, the healing process is adversely affected. Fascinated by our own technical virtuosity, we imagine that we can *fix* people, repair the body like we would repair a machine. Patient and doctor alike tend to forget the simple fact that the living body, unlike a machine has the ability to heal itself. Our best surgical techniques are in vain if wound healing is delayed or absent. Antibiotics do not control infections in the absence of body-immune response. We can create the conditions which will allow the healing process to occur, *but this autonomous healing factor is under the complete control of the psyche which, by varying its rate of vibration, can cause disease or initiate healing.* The therapeutic efficacy of any healing system is directly proportional to the patient's inner faith in that system. The stronger the faith, the faster and surer the healing.

The most important thing to know about healing is that nobody does it. You either heal yourself by stopping all ego-centered activity or you actively impede the process.

In recent years several groups have surfaced, been given credibility and flourished giving even those scientists rooted in Cartesian empiricism an opportunity to consider the "other side of the coin." The three most prominent have been the American Institute for Noetic Sciences, headed by former U.S. astronaut Dr. Edgar Mitchell, the Academy of Parapsychology and Medicine, and the Parapsychology Association which is affiliated with the American Association for the Advancement of Science (AAAS).

Our aim at the California clinic was to see if we could explore the essence of the healing process, objectively evaluate our work, and successfully apply new rituals that did not conform to current medical procedures as practiced in most hospitals, clinics, and private practices. We determined to consider the relationship between the patient's state of mind and the particular manifestation of the ailment. We felt there was some connection between mind and matter; whether consciously or unconsciously, the mind has a real influence on the type of malady, its extent, and the body's ability to heal. Perhaps, we thought, the physical symptom is a message from the body to the linear, rational, dominant hemisphere of the brain.

For a more complete description of the Lower East Side clinic see "From Suburbia to a Practice in New York Slums," *Medical World News*, May 10, 1968. The Headlands Healing Service and my association with parapsychology was developed to investigate and employ a new healing model. The essence of this model is the idea that the Cartesian approach to sciences, prevalent in medicine, has been no more effective in actual healing than have the processes Westerners have long condemned as pagan, primitive, and preposterous. Indeed, my own observations in Mexico were confirmed at a meeting in Moscow in 1972 which included physicians, biologists, physicists, psychologists, and researchers in related fields. Here was an opportunity to hear and discuss the "fields of investigation which are unexplained by the activity of the usual sense organs."

Dr. Edward Naumov, coordinator of research in the field of psychoenergetics and Director of Moscow's Institute of Technical Parapsychology, offered the above statement at the conference as a definition of *psychoenergetics*, the equivalent of the American *psi phenomena.*

While the clinic philosophy and purpose was unified, educating the patients to accept our premises was not automatic. We asked people about the nature and content of their main mental concerns at the time symptoms were first noticed. We asked simple questions like, "Are you getting enough sleep?" or "Are you perhaps drinking too much?" Many displayed anger and distrust. A typical reaction was, "Lissen, Man, I'm in here with this sore throat; didn't come in for any space rap. Just gimme some penicillin and let me get out of here."

Our average response to this was, "I'm the doctor, and it is not usual for the patient to make his own diagnosis and prescribe treatment. If you're so smart, how come you're sick?"

"Are you sure you're really a doctor?"

This phenomenon, in which the patient disassociates himself from any part in either the cause or cure of the illness, is widespread in our Western culture. People tend to cling tenaciously to their habit pattern, even in the face of violent somatic (body) opposition.

At a recent cardiology conference, it was noted that too many patients were electing to undergo coronary bypass operations for anginal chest pains rather than deal with the life-style that eventually leads to coronary disease. Most people would rather submit to an operation that promises to cure them quickly, even at the risk of death, than lose weight, give up smoking, and slow down. This is true even though the same requirements make up the program of postoperative care. Giving up work for several days of bed rest, as in the case of acute infectious disease, can precipitate a psychologic crisis. The fear of ego death is as crippling as the fear of physical death. Paradoxically, the former is a prerequisite for the cure as noted by Carl Jung, "...healing comes only from what leads the patient beyond himself and beyond his entanglement with the ego."

The Western medical model is based on the presumption that matter exists continuously in space; the organisms that contaminate and cripple the human body are outside of and are foreign to the individual. While some matter such as bacteria is detrimental to the well-being, other matter such as drugs can be utilized to reestablish health. We have accepted as fact that another individual, whose mind has become expert at the manipulation of matter, must intervene in order to dispel the disease, usually by introduction of a chemical agent. How effective is this approach?

Of all patients who consult outpatient clinical facilities in the United States, 70% are found to have no organic basis for their complaint. If the attending physician decides that the problem is mental, he either prescribes a tranquilizer or refers the patient to a psychiatrist. The remaining 30% of presenting complaints or symptoms are diseases which doctors claim exist in the body independently. The mind which inhabits the body is alleged to have no relation to or effect on the etiology and subsequent course. Within this 30% of 'real' disease, there is a group of patients who will die no matter what is done for them, and another group who get well despite medical intervention. *Those who get well because of Western medicine represent a tiny fraction of total humanity.* We must add one more group—those who die *because* of medical or surgical intervention.

In the course of a recent discussion with a young intern, the question arose as to how to treat a form of blood poisoning in which a plant, usually inhabiting the human bowel peacefully, invades the bloodstream and threatens death. When it was suggested that sonopuncture or visual imagery might be tried in addition to drugs, he responded, "That takes a lot of guts." (It seems to me that it takes more guts to medicate a patient to death. It takes less guts to try anything that might work, even though it violates the gospel of modern medical theory.)

The role of the psyche as a cause of disease or as a medium of healing is something which each individual can test out in his own living experience. I would not expect anybody to believe such a relationship exists unless they have experienced it. All one has to do is observe the events in your life in an open-minded manner. Allow that it might be true, test it out, and draw your own conclusions.

As a human, I can theoretically do anything any other human has ever been able to do. There are people who, by an act of will, can walk on hot coals without suffering burns. Under hypnosis, in controlled experiments, ordinary mortals have been able to stretch their bodies between two chairs and make them rigid enough to support the weight of another person on their abdomen. Russian experimenters have shown that yogis can cut their life processes to the point where they can exist at oxygen levels 75% below normally lethal values. The only difference between Western urban man and the Indian firewalker appears to be belief in reality. Western theology and science separates man from God, from his own physical organism, and the world in which he lives. Eastern theologies teach that divinity, body, mind and environment are all aspects of a single unitary phenomenon.

So, at one pole we have Eastern and early Gnostic Christian ideas: it's all in your mind, anything you conceive to be *out there* is an illusion. At the other pole, we find Western scientific materialism which says: it's all matter, and even your mind is just an accidental manifestation. One would like to see healing systems based on the Eastern cosmology examined dispassionately. We do not know the limitations of their theories. We do not know the limitations of a Western mind in the application of these healing techniques. We do know, as Shakespeare wrote, that "there are more things in heaven and earth, Horatio, than are dreamt of in your philosophy."

III

The reason for physical breakdown in many cases is a life pattern which does not take into account natural rhythms. The most obvious of the biologic rhythms is the diurnal (day/night) cycle. The activity of each cell in the living body varies according to the amount of solar energy available. The circadian rhythms of all body cells consist of alternating periods of activity and rest, much like the shorter rhythms of inhalation and exhalation or of cardiac systole and diastole (contraction and relaxation). The energy which powers all life processes is according to Paracelsus, transmitted as a third aspect of solar radiation; travelling through space along with heat and light, but different from either. Our ability to store this solar energy is limited. Working day and night in pursuit of ego goal exhausts available reserves and precipitates an energy crisis.

Working with students at Sonoma State College, Ruth Miller has identified four basic functions of consciousness which have approximately monthly cycles (like menstrual). These biorhythms vary in cycles covering 23 to 40 days. They seem to begin at birth and persist throughout the lifetime of the organism. Starting with the date of birth, she provides a

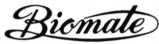
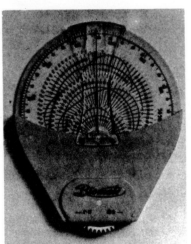
The above is one of many aids available for determining one's biorhythm activity.

computer printout of the state of efficiency of the physical (40 day), intellectual (33 day), intuitional (28 day), the emotional (23 day) functions on any given day. Japanese railroad officials keep such a record on their engineers. They have significantly reduced accidents by keeping operating personnel off the job during critical days. *All* our functions seem to operate in a cyclic on/off manner. Hospitals and surgeons are investigating the biorhythms to determine the effect they might have on the state of the patient in regard to the success or failure of the operation, and his ability to heal and recover. In due time, biorhythms may dictate the date and time of operation.

Many common diseases show a cyclic pattern. Among these are upper respiratory infections, pneumonia, and influenzas. The latter tend to recur periodically in the form of worldwide epidemics. The incidence of ulcer and asthmatic exacerbations peak sharply in the spring and fall. These are the times when the ratio of length of day to length of night is reversing. These times of polarity reversal are critical, they require a similar reversal in the activity-rest polarity of the organism. In the fall, when the days begin to grow shorter, and in the summer when the sun is high in the sky delivering greater amounts of energy over a long daily period. As fall approaches, our dose of solar energy decreases in intensity and in duration. The night power gradually becomes dominant. This is the energy of introspection, the resting phase of the annual cycle. All of nature becomes more quiescent. Man in his civilized state has lost the connection to these rhythmic events. He feels compelled to *stay in the swing* summer and winter, and continue an unremitting summer pace of activities.

At Headlands, we began to suggest to people who came into the clinic for general practice complaints (colds, diarrhea, etc.) that perhaps they should take the position of the sun into account in planning their day. We asked, "Have you considered the possibility that your illness or symptom might be a warning from your body?" The analogy of a red, oil warning light in a car was drawn. We tried to explain the dangers of being out of phase with one's own biorhythms, all to no avail. Our patients saw no reason why they couldn't be just as active in late September as they were in mid-July. A physician's function, they felt, was to prescribe the drugs which would alleviate or prevent the inevitable consequences. What they were demanding was, in essence, a pharmaceutic antidote to the rising yin power.

Scientific American recently carried a report which indicates the pineal glands of birds of some species are sensitive to light which reaches them directly through the skull. Change in light intensity or direction affects the flight pattern of blind birds. This work is important because it shows that light can affect behavior directly. We know that there are neural pathways which carry light impulses from the eye to the pineal gland in the center of the skull. Is it possible that this light is affecting and regulating our behavior? According to Dr. David Bresler of U.C.L.A., the pineal gland is the point of highest concentration of serotonin in the brain. Serotonin is the ultimate downer while norepinephrine, a relative of adrenaline, is the ultimate upper. These neurohormones are found at the point where nerve impulses must jump the gap between cells—the synapse. They regulate the rate of flow of nerve current through the body.

Consider the change which comes over any group of living creatures when the sun comes out after a prolonged rainstorm. The sudden burst of solar energy initiates sharply increased activity. During the period of darkness and rain we tend to be more quiet and subdued. Many consider themselves to be depressed or moody, forgetting the connection between the state of mind and the state of weather.

The sun is not the only extra terrestial power source which affects our behavior and mental state. About 10 years ago I attended a lecture at New York's Hayden Planetarium. The speaker, a physicist from the Massachusetts Institute of Technology, was discussing quasars, then a newly discovered source of energy radiation in deep space. He explained that these quasistellar radio sources seem to exist at the outer limits of our known universe. They represent points in deep space which are capable of radiating huge amounts of energy over short periods of time. The particular source under consideration gives off energy bursts in the order of thirty trillion suns over a period of twenty-four earth hours. Scientists at M.I.T. were interested in correlating events on our planet with these cataclysmic cosmic episodes. Data was fed into computers from quasar C236. Results indicated that the energy would have reached our solar system on Black Tuesday in 1929, the day of the stock market crash which marked the beginning of world-wide depression and rocked the entire civilized world. There *seems to be* a definite temporal relationship between social and cosmic events in this case at least. Other sources of cosmic energy include the center of our own galaxy, which is known to emit huge bursts of radiation intermittently, exploding solar systems, and radiation from neighboring extragalactic sources.

How might such influences affect individual consciousness? Sudden unexplained changes in mood might be one way. Things might be going along smoothly, when the consciousness seems to be seized from outside, as it were, by a tightness in the chest, a knot in the stomach, or a vague feeling of malaise. At this point, one tends to look around for someone on whom to blame it. This is usually husband, wife, boss, or anyone else who happens to be handy. Looking for a reason, many people spend huge amounts of time and money in the pursuit of obscure childhood trauma. Carl Jung notes that in cases of argument between husband and wife each thinks the situation is unique. He points out that this same exchange has taken place in innumerable languages, in innumerable human groups since time began. He suggests that the causes transcend the individual and his personal relationships. If you observe yourself carefully next time you get a knot in your stomach, you will find that the feeling comes first, then you begin to search for reasons in the past or in the immediate environment. Failing to find such a reason, an honest individual may say, "I don't know what came over me." The loss of control could just as easily be caused by the explosion of a solar system.

An energy burst reaching us from the galactic center is an event described by the male, linear cerebral hemisphere, the thinker. The left cerebral hemisphere, the conscious domain relies on the unconscious to store information. Medical research has split the brain in two in a breakthrough which

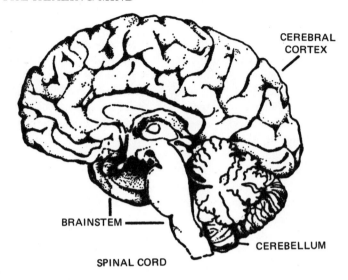

CEREBRAL CORTEX

BRAINSTEM

CEREBELLUM

SPINAL CORD

SECTION VIEW FROM LEFT OF BRAIN

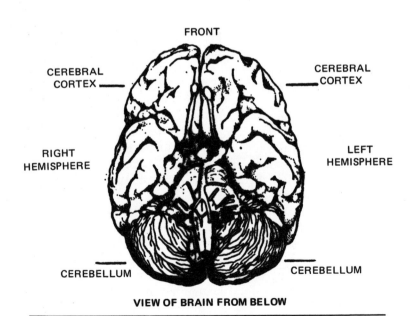

FRONT

CEREBRAL CORTEX

CEREBRAL CORTEX

RIGHT HEMISPHERE

LEFT HEMISPHERE

CEREBELLUM

CEREBELLUM

VIEW OF BRAIN FROM BELOW

TWO VIEWS OF THE BRAIN

rivals the physicist's discovery of atomic fission. In confirmation of the writings of giants like Freud and Jung we are now being told that our cerebral hemispheres constitute two separate brains. Only the dominant hemisphere which houses the speech center is connected to our consciousness. The activities of the subdominant hemisphere which concerns itself with spatial relationships and visual imagery are usually repressed or ignored.

The diagram below shows the divisions of the brain and their related functions.

The peripheral nervous system is seen to be divided according to classical concepts into the autonomic system and the craniospinal system. The central nervous system is divided into the archipallium below the old brain that man shares with the other vertebrates, and the neopallium above the new brain whose most significant development is in man, dolphins notwithstanding.

UNCONSCIOUS DOMAIN	CONSCIOUS DOMAIN
1. archipallium, in the central nervous system	1. neopallium, in the central nervous system
2. Control of smooth muscle and glands in the automatic section of the peripheral nervous system	2. control of striate muscle in the craniospinal section of the peripheral nervous system
3. involuntary	3. voluntary
4. responsive to "passive volition"	4. responsive to "active volition"

The dashed line, the divider between conscious and unconscious systems and processes, is drawn as a straight line, but it is to be visualized as a continuously undulating boundary between conscious and unconscious processes and brain structures, as *attention* shifts from one brain region to another. For instance, when one learns to drive a car many of the at-first-conscious striate muscular activities upon which much attention is lavished gradually become unconscious, and eventually it is possible when the mind is preoccupied to drive through miles of traffic without awareness of other cars or traffic signals.

On the other hand, the involuntary nervous system is not necessarily "involuntary," even as the voluntary system is not necessarily "voluntary." If we concentrate attention on our right hand for a few seconds, its temperature will spontaneously begin to rise or fall due to tensing or relaxing of smooth muscles embedded in blood vessel walls, depending among other things on our previous conditioning to self-examination. After training in temperature control, however, many subjects can increase or decrease the volume of blood in the hands at will. Consciousness of the specific neural pattern involved is *not* obtained, however, any more than there is consciousness of the neural network in the voluntary nervous system that causes the arm to move from side to side "at will"; in both cases, autonomic (automatic) and craniospinal (willed), the desired behavior is obtained through visualization of the desired event accompanied by volition. The significant difference in controlling these two systems is that for the control of the voluntary nervous system it is necessary to use *active* volition, and for control of the involuntary nervous system it is necessary to use *passive* volition. This last sounds like a contradiction in terms. How can anyone have passive volition? Passive volition might best be described as detached effortless volition.

The psychophysiological principle affirms that every change in the mental-emotional state, conscious or unconscious, is accompanied by an appropriate change in the physiologic state and, conversely, every change in the physiologic state reflects a change in the mental-emotional state. This closed Newtonian type of principle, when coupled with volition, which is at least at present of indeterminate origin, makes possible a psychosomatic self-regulation. Whether volition has origin beyond the physiological matrix as a metaforce is the essence of the mind-body problem. [9]

The somatic body is one route by which the subdominant cerebral hemisphere communicates with you. It is the source of the body image—the mediatrix of biofeedback from the body to the left-sided, conscious mind. It is through physical disease that we all *suffer the slings and arrows* of an outraged subconscious. Ease, as opposed to disease, may be seen as a state of harmonious equilibrium between the two equipotent, autonomous, cerebral hemispheres one of which is conscious (sun, yang, male), and one of which is subconscious (moon, yin, female). If contact is established between the two hemispheres (the alchemical mystical marriage), healing energy (the panacea) is released. The healing energy is the same as the energy tied up in the symptom (the *prima materia*).

The separation of the two hemispheres was successfully demonstrated in an ingenious experiment with patients in whom the connecting fibers between the two brain halves were cut as a result of a disease process. A group of several common objects was placed on the table before the person being tested. He focused his gaze at a point in front of him in such a manner that he could still see the objects on the table. The word for one of the things on the table was flashed into the nasal side of his left eye for a small fraction of a second. This subliminal impulse was carried to his feminine right cerebral hemisphere. If, for instance, the word *key* was flashed into the nasal half of his left eye, he would reach out with his left hand and pick up the key. The right hemisphere controls the left side of the body.

Why did he select the key? In each trial, the man was totally unaware of the fact that his left hand had reached out and selected a particular object from the table. He was also totally unaware of the fact that he had received a subliminal command to his right hemisphere to perform this specific action in space. His subconscious (right cerebral hemisphere) had received and carried out the command independently from and without the knowledge of his left hemispheric, dominant, conscious mind.

The right cerebral hemisphere, the female, makes the pictures we call dreams, hallucinations, mental images or empirical reality depending on the bias of our particular society. The left cerebral hemisphere, the male side, names and classifies images. Both are processing cosmic energy in opposite modes, yin and yang. Between the hemispheres, and below them in the brain lies the hypothalamus, and the old brain which we share with lower forms of life. This structure runs all the automatic processes in the body. It is a bio-computer. It monitors and regulates heart rate, blood pressure, chemical balance, and every vital function you don't have to think about. It is also the seat of the emotions which it creates and regulates through a complex network of nerves and hormones. Receiving impulses from both cerebral hemispheres, it converts information into bodily states (as in the fight-or-flight reaction, or sexual arousal). It also controls the body's system of defense. This magnificent computer is controlled and programmed by the cerebral cortical brain, consciously or unconsciously. *Cancer, arthritis, heart disease, and stroke are likely to be bodily states induced by an unconscious command or picture of self-destruction.* The female, form-creating hemisphere contains the body image. It communicates by means of unconscious gestures, smiles, frowns, raised eyebrows, and the like. Since it shares control over the body through the hypothalamic computer, perhaps it can induce healing in case of faulty programming or disease.

"According to medical specialists, perhaps as much as 80% of human problems involve psychosomatic disease, either totally or as a contributing factor...this means ...that a certain section of the brain ...the right hemisphere, learned a bad habit ...and is functioning in an undesirable manner. Research is showing that these bad habits can be voluntarily eliminated by retraining, using biofeedback to tell us what is happening in the physiological domain so that we can become aware of, and use, specific existential changes that are correlated with specific physiological changes. It seems reasonable to assume that if we can get physiologically sick from responding psychologically to stress in some inappropriate way, we can perhaps get well by learning to control the physiologic response. Feedback devices are important for this kind of learning because they mirror what is going on beneath the skin. Visual feedback tells us when our car is going off the road; biofeedback tells us about our bodies and allows us to make existential corrections." [10]

IV

One of the early workers in the field of biofeedback was Dr. Neal Miller of New York's Rockefeller University. Orthodox medical opinions until recently held that the idea of being able to control our own involuntary processes (heart rate, blood pressure, bleeding, healing, etc.) was ridiculous. For this reason, Dr. Miller had trouble getting laboratory space and student assistance. Despite non-cooperation, he developed the techniques of biofeedback. This is a means by which modern technology performs the marriage between the conscious and the unconscious minds. He proved that the conscious mind can command the unconscious to restore bodily functions to normal. "We are now able to regard the activities of our internal organs as behavior in the same sense that the movements of our hands and fingers are behavior."

In order to control automatic behavior, we must become aware of what that behavior *feels* like, or looks like. We must establish sensory contact with the part or function of the body we are trying to affect. In the case of high blood pressure, a device is rigged which flashes a light or sounds a buzzer when the pressure drops. The patient concentrates on making the buzzer buzz in the same manner as one tries to control the course of a pinball or a bowling ball—by an act of concentrated will. A significant number of patients cause the buzzer to buzz, and their blood pressure falls to normal. At Bellevue Hospital in New York, people who have been paralyzed were treated with biofeedback techniques. (Insofar as they wed a conscious with an unconscious process, they must also be considered alchemical techniques.) An electromyograph, which converts muscle contraction into an electric signal, was the connecting medium. Muscle contraction was unconscious because the sensory nerve to the extremity had been severed or injured. The electric signal from the EMG is used to make the buzzer sound. This replaces the nerve in that it makes the contraction of the muscle observable by the conscious mind. A flashing light accomplishes the same purpose. "See the light flashing, command it to do so with your conscious mind."

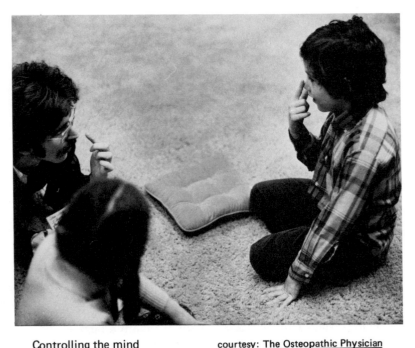

Controlling the mind   courtesy: <u>The Osteopathic Physician</u>

In December 1971, Dr. Herbert F. Johnson of Casa Colima Hospital for Rehabilitative Medicine in Pomona, California, reported that this technique helped some of his crippled patients walk without braces after only a few weeks' work. By reestablishing sensory connection with a paralyzed limb, it was possible to regain voluntary control.

If you can't feel a limb, you can't move it. Tensing the muscles tells us where the limb is. Dr. J. Brundy of the New York University Medical Center noted, "There is no motor performance unless there is sensory feedback and instantaneous confirmation. Perhaps these people could learn control of muscles if we supplied an external feedback loop through the senses of sight and hearing..."

Working with a 24-year-old man with a broken neck who was a total care patient, Dr. Brundy helped him to the point where he can operate an electric wheelchair, eat a sandwich, shave, and smoke a cigarette. He can make the muscle move by causing the light to flash. Once this is accomplished and consolidated, the machine is no longer required. "You know," says Dr. Brundy, "that's very meaningful for a guy who has spent three years on his back without being able to scratch his nose." College students were trained at the Menninger Clinic to produce *theta reverie*. This is a state in which the buzzer was made to sound when the brain produced 4-7 cycles per second on the EEG (electroencephalograph). In this vibratory range, there appear "hypnagogic images which come right up out of the unconscious" according to Dr. Elmer Green. The students could either watch the images while they were fully awake, or they could ask them their significance to the questioner's daily life. The answer seems to flash into the querant's mind as if the mental image itself were responding. It is possible that the mental image may provide an internal biofeedback loop between the conscious left hemispheric ego and the diseased or misbehaving somatic organism. Carl Jung refers to these imaginary figures as "...psychic projections which bring unconscious contents to light, often in the form of vivid visions." They have their origin in the form-making right hemisphere.

Modern society teaches us to repress relentlessly the images flashed to us by the subdominant hemisphere. In these circumstances, Dr. Jung feels, "... the unconscious (hemisphere) has, as it were, no alternative but to generate... (physical disease)...and neurotic symptoms." In theta reverie and similar states, we work on the borders of consciousness so as to induce that which is unconscious, (the conflicting manifesting as the symptom) to cross the threshold and come within our reach.

The autonomous image, projected by the nonverbal feminine hemisphere mediates between the left-brained ego and the right hemisphere's body image. As the representative of the unconscious, the image has the ability to translate the message of the symptoms into a linear, verbal form. Establishment of a dialogue between the patient and his vision seems to expedite healing.

The alchemists, the Buddhists, and the Egyptian hermetic physicians considered that they had discovered the secret of healing. All their methods require that the disciple get quiet enough to begin to hallucinate. This was often accomplished by periods of up to 20 years of sensory deprivation, either in a cave, a cell, or in the desert. These same images appear spontaneously as dreams, even to the uninitiated. Drugs like LSD, marijuana, and alcohol strongly stimulate the flow of mental imagery, overpowering the thinker in the left brain.

The left hemisphere thinker can be put at rest by a variety of techniques. These have by and large been formalized as religious rituals, hypnotic suggestions, or sensory deprivation, among others. Another way to shift the balance in favor of the image-making brain is to overload the thinker. The Buddhists give him an insoluble problem like, "What is the sound of one hand clapping?" This is called a *koan*. If the thinker is quiescent or overloaded to the point of exhaustion, energy flows through the body according to the prevailing pattern of the cosmos, precipitating as healthy tissue—this prevents the onset of disease.

Confirmation of the validity of ancient models comes from Dr. Robert Ornstein of the Langley Porter Neuropsychiatric Institute in San Francisco. The normal brain constantly exhibits electrical activity in the form of very low voltages as recorded at the scalp by the EEG. If this activity is in the range of four to twelve cycles/second, it is called the *alpha state.* This signal represents a carrier wave much like the 60-cycle hum emitted by a turned on, but inactive, transmitter. A person involved in a verbal task such as writing a shopping list, tends to turn off the female side of the brain. The same person trying to picture a living room, shuts off the male side of consciousness, emitting alpha waves from the left hemisphere. The living room exists in two aspects: a pair of words as spoken by the male cerebral hemisphere, and a picture flashed by the female counterpart. Dr. Ornstein feels that in daily life we tend to alternate between a verbal and a pictorial world, varying the balance according to the situation.

"The appearance of the alpha rhythm indicates a turning off of information processing in the area involved. As if to reduce the interference between the two conflicting modes of operation of its two cerebral hemispheres, the brain tends to turn off its unused side in a given situation." If you turn off your thoughts, your external reality tends to disappear. If you get comfortable, relax your body, and stop thinking, the world begins to dissolve, as in sleep. It may be replaced by a dream world which seems at the time equally real and substantial. Carl Jung believes that the two worlds have their origin in one source, the psyche or the self. The self is hermaphroditic. Each one of us is two individuals, a male and female. The former is rational, can speak and think thoughts. The female side makes the pictures, dreams, mental images, and empirical reality.

We must seriously consider the possibility that works like the Cabala (a Jewish system of theosophy which centers on the belief in creation through emanation) and the Upanishad (ancient Hindu philosophy based on one ultimate reality) were cosmologies based on the theories of highly evolved scientific minds. Cro-Magnon man is 35,000 years old, his technologic achievements (like the Great Pyramid at Gizeh or the recently discovered crystal skull) surpass the capability of our modern technology. A California state textbook, *Early Man,* tells us they produced "the first art...sculptures, paintings and stone engravings so powerfully conceived and executed as to rank among mankind's great artistic achievements." Physically modern man differs little from Cro-Magnon man; what sets the two apart is culture. Actually, Jung says the two exist together in each one of us—a modest enough observation.

Taoist philosophers tell us that the entire manifested universe is created by the struggle and interplay between light and dark forces. Each contains and engenders the other. Eastern mystics, ancient Cabalists, and Western particle physicists agree on an axiom of cosmogenesis. They all agree that there can be no manifestation without differentiation into a pair of opposites. In the laboratory this concept is confirmed by the observation that in high velocity particle collisions, no particle splits into less than two oppositely charged subparticles. Any pair of opposites then, represents two aspects of the primal entity whose division created them.

The Egyptian physicians referred to the right cerebral hemisphere (form-creating and feminine) as *Isis*, the Cabalists called it *Binah*. Binah and Chockmah, the left cerebral hemisphere, make up *Kether*, totality. Kether is said to emanate from the *limitless light*. The light is equivalent to consciousness in practically every human cosmology, as when we refer to a radical and significant increase in our conscious understanding as *seeing the light*. The Cabala clearly intimates by its arrangement of the cosmic *tree of life* that consciousness creates the brain which manifests in two complementary halves. The Chinese also present us with a model of human consciousness and its trinitarian structure.

Do you suppose that when St. John had his apocalyptic vision of the New Jerusalem as a city with twelve gates or when the authors of the New Testament recorded that Christ (the light, consciousness) was served by twelve apostles they were aware of the fact that the human brain (the seat of consciousness), is served by twelve pairs of cranial nerves? These nerves (apostles, gates) form the connecting link between consciousness and the world *out there*. Is the Cabala an anatomic and psychiatric treatise on the nature of human consciousness, or is Gray's *Anatomy* a mystical exercise? Is it indeed possible that each is describing the same phenomenon in its own terms? St. John's vision originated, according to the most modern view of the phenomenon of consciousness, in his female cerebral hemisphere.

The ancients believed that the key to wholeness (healing) lay in the mental image. In order to induce formation of the mental image, it is necessary to go into a meditative state which turns off the thinker. When the left hemisphere is at rest or in alpha, it is possible to reprogram the computer by means of the conscious image of the healthy state. According to our working theory, this image is transmitted holographically and reproduced in the matter of the body. The image is the junction point of the four aspects of human psychic experience—totality: male and female conscious and unconscious.

Astrology tells us that there are four cardinal signs; we divided the year into four seasons, the earth into four quarters. The number four as an indicator of totality has appeared in human dreams, visions, art, religion, mythology, and fairy tales since the beginning of recorded time. The totality of consciousness has four aspects. Dr. Jung suggests that they are thinking, feeling, sensing, and intuiting. This last is a statement of his dominant, male linear, left cerebral hemisphere. The same intuitive knowledge is flashed to consciousness in the form of the vision of the four angles around the throne of God (St. John) or of the four cherubim which defined the center of the vision of Ezekiel. We call the left hemispheric linear, verbal arrangement of data, science. This same information programmed and projected in symbols and mirages onto the back of our eyeballs by the feminine right hemisphere, is repressed as mysticism at best, lunacy at worst.

At the clinic during our early sonopuncture experiment we had an experience of the spontaneous image projection that supported the hypothesis of four-part totality. The patient was the short-order cook in the local restaurant-pool hall. Mostly he likes cooking, baseball, and staying stoned. The Sunday baseball games are a tradition of sorts. Jimmy's greatest accomplishment was taking part in the game where the local *heads* got stoned and played the *greasers* (young conservatives) who were straight. The *heads* won, but in the course of the game our patient was struck over the right eyebrow by a stinging line drive. He has sustained a laceration over the acupuncture point *bladder 2.* He had had adequate medical treatment for the laceration the previous day. His complaint was, "I just feel spaced out all the time." He appeared extremely tense and moved constantly in a manner suggesting agitation. When we asked him about this he responded, "Yeah, Man, I'm freaked."

He attributed his agitated, sleepless state to the after-effects of the blow. In the course of examination, it was noted that there was moderate swelling at the site of a cut over the acupuncture point. Touching the area around the acupuncture point caused the patient to shriek loudly as his entire body shuddered convulsively. The bladder meridian is a yang meridian. We reasoned that perhaps this state of unnatural excitement was related to continued stimulation of that meridian by the blow and the subsequent swelling. A beam of high frequency sound was directed into the bladder meridian on the outside of his right ankle. Ten minutes after treatment he had completely regained his composure and was offering free lunch for two as an expression of his gratitude. That night he had a dream in which he saw an equal-armed cross dividing a circle into four quarters. He had no idea what the dream meant, but he felt it was very important and that it made him feel really good.

The circle, the equal-armed cross, and the concept of four are all symbols of totality or wholeness. To heal means to make whole. Dr. Jung believed that these images have the power to initiate healing without the cooperation or knowledge of the intellect. The image's power to heal is measured by its numinousity, its power to arouse emotion. The stronger the energy charge in the image, the stronger the emotion aroused. This is an indication of the degree to which the energy outflow from the right side of the brain is running over to stimulate the hypothalamus and the endrocrine system. The sight of Old Glory, for instance, can make a patriot's heart swell with pride. A rapidly moving electron beam can drive him into acute agitation and fury if it creates on his TV screen the image of a protestor burning his flag. This same image could enter the consciousness of a disinterested foreign observer without setting off his endocrines, without getting his juices flowing, so to speak.

In the first case, the image of the burning symbol (the flag), like a real tiger, sets off the fight or flight alarm reaction. It does this without consulting the left hemispheric intellect. The part which says I, for its part, feels itself seized by urges and moods which it cannot control. These urges and moods are mediated by the body. I can control them only with difficulty if at all. The body image lies in the right cerebral hemisphere. Connections with the hypothalamus cause violent bodily changes, "I don't know what came over me," says the speech center.

An image can also convert a symptom into a message from the feminine unconscious to the masculine thinker. This is because each represents a different aspect or form of a single energy. Using this approach, we ask our patients to think of the ache or symptom in terms of bioplasmic energy which is now flowing freely through the body meridians. In order to deal with the symptom, its energy must be transformed into a usable form. It is not possible to destroy energy, we can only change its form. A repressed symptom always pops up somewhere else with increased virulence. It is like a ringing telephone which persists in signaling until there is a response. *The cause of an illness is not removed with the suppression of the symptom.* This approach robs us of a valuable signpost pointing to the cause; which is invariably a state of mind. It may represent a conflict between the male and female halves of our conscious unity. An illness indicates that the patient is engaged in an activity which is in conflict with his deepest needs and/or desires. Isis, the feminine hemisphere, signals the computer in the hypothalamus to create a body state which reflects the conflict. It is through the body image that she communicates with her conscious counterpart, Osiris, the masculine hemisphere. She can also create moods and project dreams and visions. If you have the physical or mental symptom, you have created it in your female hemisphere in order to tell yourself something. In order to get the message it is necessary to suspend activity of the male hemisphere; this is called meditation.

Transcendental meditation "apparently induces a hypo-metabolic (less than normal life processes) state during alert wakefulness," according to Dr. David W. Doner, Jr., assistant chief of the renal section at the Boston Veterans Administration Hospital. During meditation, he noted, respiratory rate and volume fall; pulse and heart rate slow; forearm blood flow increases; blood lactate decreases rapidly and steeply; electrical skin resistance rises. It seems to affect every organ system in the body!

Meditators sit quietly, eyes closed, for twenty minutes twice a day, a relaxation technique that is easily learned and that requires little effort, according to Dr. Doner. During meditation, the EEG shows intensification of slow alpha waves at 8 or 9 cycles/second in the frontal and central portions of the brain. He has also noted greater integration of the right and left brains.

Dr. Patricia Carrington, Lecturer in the Department of Psychology at Princeton University, described TM as "A reconditioning of my central nervous system. Within about ten days of learning to meditate, I stopped having an intense startle response and no longer had a sense of muscular tightening every time there was a trivial accident."

After utilizing meditation in the treatment of 34 patients, Dr. Carrington reported: "In many there was tension reduction, a lessening of anxiety and disappearance of inappropriate startle responses. The decrease in overreaction to frustration can be quite dramatic and can markedly improve interpersonal relationships. We noticed also an improvement in such psychosomatic conditions as tension headaches. We see in many patients a general energy release, with increased physical stamina, or a lessened need for daytime naps, and increased productivity."

In our experiments at the clinic, we ask the patient to picture himself in a comfortable and safe place. He is told to sit quietly in his imaginary workshop and watch. In a room, a door will open; in the country, someone or something will appear on a path. When the figure appears, ask it, "Are you the one who created the symptoms?" In case of an affirmative answer, the apparition is asked to clarify the importance of the illness. At this point in the procedure, our patients either smile broadly or laugh out loud. The response always tells the patient what was done in his personal life to cause the illness, and precisely what must be done to get rid of it. One patient was told by his image, a wise old man, "You're not centered, you need to be alone more."

V

"Do you think acupuncture could help diabetes? I've had it for twenty-five years." He says he is thirty-five, but he looks ten years younger. He shoots 40 units of insulin twice daily, and his name is Barry.

"I have to get a physical every six months for my job; I see only the best doctors...you ever hear of the Joslin Clinic?"

Dressed in sneakers, brown pants, and a white tee shirt, he notes that in the current literature on acupuncture, there is no reference to the treatment of diabetes. "I've been going through some real heavy changes these past two weeks... whenever I start to think about my job, my blood sugar goes up, and I have to take more insulin; then I calm down, and I start to go into shock. They say I'm a 'brittle diabetic' (my blood sugar bounces around a lot). It seems to be connected to my thought content. Last year I started thinking about arthritis, and the joints in my wrists and hands began to swell and hurt. They came back to normal only after I stopped thinking I had arthritis."

As he squats on the grass, someone notes the Tibetan contention that 'when thoughts cease, phenomena cease.' Emblazoned on the front of his white tee shirt is the figure of a crowned hermaphrodite; half man, half woman, with the white male face and figure facing to Barry's right, and the dark female part of the single body facing left. "It's a Jung tee shirt; I got real compulsive about wearing it...I wear it all the time."

The steeple of the Calvary Presbyterian Church cuts the scene in two, duplicating the symbol on the tee shirt. To the East, the clinic yard bakes in the bright September sun. The western half lies in the cool, dark steeple shadow. Barry chooses to remain in the shade. "Dr. Carl Jung, the famous shrink."

He understands that our technique is related to acupuncture and he would sure like to see if it would help his diabetes as he is getting real tired of it. He cannot get himself to believe that his affliction is nothing more than a crystalization of his thought patterns, but seems willing to consider the possibility. An electrical engineer by training, he is now looking into silk-screening. Our approach to this patient must satisfy the scientist as well as the artist if it is to have any hope for success. Healing requires a 'heiros gamos' (mystical marriage) between the two opposing aspects of Barry's personality. He will arrange for his treating physician to send records and monitor his progress.

The standard treatment for diabetes hasn't changed since I got out of medical school in 1955. This treatment has not demonstrably altered the course of the disease nor has it, in the past 20 years shown any effect on the development of vascular and other sequelae (complications). We achieve temporary relief by repeatedly plunging a hollow steel spike into the arm, thigh or abdomen of the victim; every day, for as *long* as he lives.

The theory out of which this marginally successful treatment evolved states that diabetes mellitus occurs when the Islands of Langerhans stop production and shipment of insulin. Why do these cells in the pancreas suddenly shut down and die? Well, no one knows for sure, but the result is a buildup in the bloodstream of chemical poisons called ketone bodies. These along with unburned sugar accumulate in the blood and spill over into the urine. When the level of poisons is high enough, there is an interruption of consciousness and the patient is said to be in diabetic coma. If we regularly inject insulin into the body, we can, in many cases, control hyperglycemia (high blood sugar) and ketosis (accumulation of ketone bodies).

At this point, it would be well to take note of an observation by Albert Einstein; 'Physical concepts are free creations of the human mind and not, however it may seem, uniquely determined by the external world.' We may, if we like, freely create the concept that Barry's diabetes, like his arthritis, was created and maintained by his thought pattern. If he could establish contact with his pancreas, he might be able to command it to produce insulin. He might also work on changing his customary thought pattern or see if he could control it to the point where his thoughts cease. About once a week we will direct a beam of ultra sound, vibrating at a rate of 1 million cycles/second into his appropriate acupuncture points. Our concept is useless to Barry unless it helps him eliminate his dependence on externally administered insulin. He wants to kick his habit, so to speak.

The following day Aphrodite comes in, looks around, and seats herself on a couch in the waiting room. Her name is Sarah and she is interested in working in the field of parapsychology. For the past nine months she has been living on money she accumulated working as a cocktail waitress at Tahoe.

"I own a house, and this guy I'm living with makes the payments; I have no trouble finding work, I get any regular job I ever apply for." (It is easy to see why.) She is 33, has been to college, and was told nine months ago that she had cancer of the cervix.

"When I refused to let him cut it out, this surgeon told me that I had an unnatural attachement to my uterus." She quit her job and gave full time to her meditation in which she pictured a 'normal healthy, beautiful uterus.' "The cancer disappeared. When I went back to the doctor and told him how I did it, he said I was crazy."

Mother Earth, barefoot, tent-like cotton dress covering her huge frame, agrees to let Sarah look in on her treatment.

She spent a good deal of time in India, and is a disciple of Sri Aurobindo. She undertook a series of sonopuncture treatments to see if she could lose some weight. "I tell you, that sound acupuncture stuff is transcendental medication. It takes me to a level of cellular consciousness. I am no longer aware of my gross physical body, time or space. I have no sense of being a person. I completely forget where I am and I lose all sense of time." Josie takes her treatment in the lotus position with her eyes closed. Sarah recognizes the state of rapture. She quotes an old Bengali text which describes it. "The self is void, the world is void; heaven, earth and the space between are void." Another young woman described the same experience during sonopuncture. Her brain waves which were being monitored showed an increase in alpha (8-12 cycles/second) rhythm. Yogis in deep trance also show a predominance of alpha waves. Sex is a common vehicle for attaining this particular state of consciousness. In his *Masks of God: Creative Mythology*, Joseph Campbell notes that, "As though struck by lightning, so is one by love, which is a divine seizure, transmuting the life, erasing every interfering thought."

The ability to achieve ecstasy (standing outside space, time, ego, and the physical body) seems to exert a profoundly beneficial effect on the health and well being of the human organism. Before I can evolve into someone else, I must relinquish all that I am now. I must shed my identity like a snake sheds it's skin; periodically in order to accommodate the inexorable process of growth and change. 'Those dead, who are not dead but sleep' need to note the fact that we are now entering the last quarter of the twentieth century. The turn of the century marks radical changes in society's dominant physical concepts; our view of what constitutes reality.

Mid-twentieth century medical science built a picture of the human body which was based largely on observation of lifeless cadavers. The tissues to be studied are cut away from the whole, imbedded in wax after drying them out; stained, and examined under a microscope which magnifies up to 440 times. On the basis of this archaic procedure the wife of an American president agreed to have one breast and a large portion of the flesh constituting her chest hacked away.

Following this disfigurement, she was informed that there was a 40% chance that she would die within the next five years, anyway. Upon reading press accounts of the grisly affair, thousands of women hurried to have breast examinations: presumably to see if they too could qualify for radical surgery. As in the case of diabetes, the treatment for cancer of the breast has neither improved nor changed significantly over the past twenty years. The president's lady, unlike Sarah, did not suffer from neurotic attachement to the specifically feminine parts of her anatomy. Like Barry, she consulted the best doctors, and following their advice, sacrificed the flesh of her living body on the sterile stainless steel altar of a healing cult which blindly accepts an outmoded, discredited, mechanistic view of physical reality.

Humanity has a right to demand more from those entrusted with the task of alleviating suffering and the ravages of disease. The October 14, 1974 issue of *Time* magazine documents the bankruptcy of the twentieth century medical model when it observes "Despite the widespread occurrence of breast cancer (300,000 deaths and 90,000 new cases this year) its treatment remains in dispute." "The common procedure... is a radical mastectomy, a disfiguring and sometimes partially disabling operation that involves removal of the breast, the underlying pectoral muscle and the lymphatic tissue under the arm... The operation...can produce lifelong pain, weakness and periodic swelling in the affected arm."

Three to five days after the ritual dismemberment, a severe depression usually sets in. A fifty-one-year old victim says, "I felt shattered, ashamed...degraded." The operating surgeons do not usually concern themselves with this aspect of the disaster. This is often left to volunteers who offer 'practical advice on where to buy bras and prostheses.' "We can also help them to understand that breasts do not make a woman," notes the female coordinator of one such group.

Humanity has a right to demand more.

Joseph was born in 1910. A botanist, he said that his intense interest in living plants had made him an expert, provided him with a livelihood, and caused him ten years of unremitting pain and disability. Standing on crutches because 'it hurts just as much whether I sit or stand' he explained that his hip joint had been eaten away at the upper lip and his second lumbar vertabra had collapsed. The cause for this destructive arthritis was a rare infection by a form of Brucellosis (B. Souis). He had contracted it digging in a pile of infected compost. It had already killed two of his colleagues who were similarly infected. He was taking up to three grains of codeine daily to keep his pain within tolerable limits. At the beginning, only injected morphine gave him relief, but he had cut it out of the management of his disease for fear of becoming addicted. His therapeutic goal is 'relief of this damned pain,' and the ability to go about one-half mile up a hillside to get a rare wildflower specimen. He had been to the best doctors and they seemed unable to relieve his pain or to find a way to impede the inexorable decline in his physical condition. "Oh, yes," he noted, "I also have high blood pressure...they can't help that either."

The energy source in our experiment with Joseph was mechanical vibration induced in a quartz crystal through the piezo-electric effect. Vibratory energy at a frequency of one million cycles/second was delivered to the patient's acupuncture system, through an air tight medium. (Glycerin or mineral oil are excellent.) The sonic generator used in this case is commonly found in the offices of physiotherapists and of physicians. It is simple to use, harmless, and relatively cheap. It is commonly called an ultra sound machine. A beam of ultra sound was directed into Joseph's acupuncture system through six points for 1-2 minutes per point at an intensity of 0.4 to 0.6 watts/sq. cm. Ten minutes after the treatment, he was able to walk ten feet across the waiting room without his crutches. He had not been able to do this for ten years.

A week later, Joseph reported that he was completely pain free for the first time in ten years. For a period of four days following the treatment, he took no pain pills. He has also been able to walk one-eighth of a mile without crutches.

Our own clinical work at the Headlands, along with the reports cited, might lead one to postulate that *Non-specific stimulation of human acupuncture points relieve the suffering of acute pain due to various causes.*

As a general practitioner, in face to face relationship with Joseph the human, I am committed to helping him achieve his therapeutic goal by any means. I don't really know if the treatment closed a gate in the spinal cord, or if it ironed out standing waves in a fourth human circulatory system, or if it did anything at all, since there were other factors in his treatment regimen. I do know that my patient improved, felt better, and made rapid and obvious progress toward a therapeutic goal he had himself selected. If absolute reality is impossible to determine, the physician must remain a pragmatist and apply only those theories which get clinical results. He must quickly and simply alleviate pain and suffering. It is conceivable in the light of present scientific thought that *all* our therapeutic procedures are nothing more than ritual, no more effective than cookbook acupuncture or cookbook alchemy. The theoretical justification for a clinical procedure must take second place to its therapeutic efficacy.

Recognizing the developing detente between modern science and alchemy, the physician must reexamine and reevaluate medicine's alchemical roots. The concept of psychosomatic disease holds that problems such as asthma, allergy, and perhaps cancer itself are as much psychical as they are physical. We may hypothesize that any physical state is as much a reflection of the state of the physical matter of the body as it is a reflection of the psyche which inhabits the body.

Joseph has a 300-year-old Indian healing stone. Following the instruction of the medicine man who presented it to him, he places it over his hip and directs healing energy through the amulet into the ailing joint. "Cement head" cosmology relegates this procedure to the realm of occult quackery because there is no connection they can see between the healing stone and the physical matter of the degenerating bone. Galileo, using the same reasoning, dismissed as occult nonsense the idea that the moon was able to affect the tidal behavior of earth's oceans across the empty vastness of space. Today's physics postulates that gravity, one of four basic forces in nature is mediated through the action of 'gravitons.' Gravitons are said to be vibrations in a non-medium called the 'psi field.'

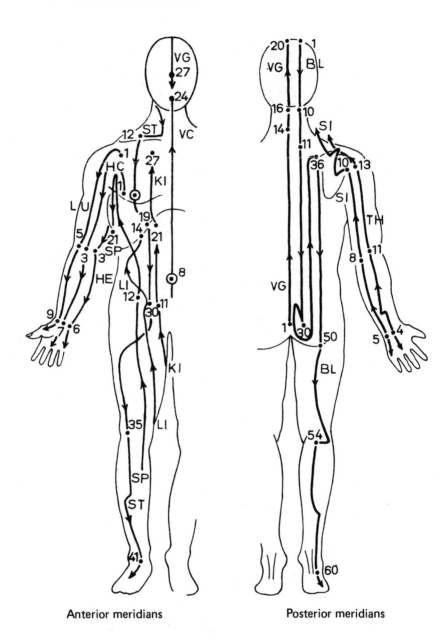

Anterior meridians   Posterior meridians

POINTS OF CHINESE ACUPUNCTURE

In this respect they resemble electrons or protons which behave like waves in the hypothetical 'psi field' when they are not acting like discrete particles in space. Directed conscious attention may be seen as a congruent beam of wave-particles called 'mindons' which like gravitons travel through empty space as waves in the psi field and exert a visible effect on particulate matter. Directed attention may provide a non-specific stimulus which can affect the activity of the acupuncture points. Investigations in this area continue in the United States, Russia, and Germany as well as in other countries. This research offers promise of a breakthrough in the healing arts equivalent to the discovery of penicillin or anesthetics.

Einstein told us that matter and energy are two faces of a unity. Wolfgang Pauli sees mind and body as two aspects of a single process. Freud contributed the observation that a great portion of this process is outside our awareness in a space he called 'the unconscious.' Invisible and unknown to our waking thoughts, the Jungian 'unconscious' includes everything in the universe which is not contained in the waking mind. That's just about everything there is! The unconscious, according to the theories of Freud and Jung, controls and directs human life experience almost completely. Insofar as the conscious mind does not concern itself with them, all vital bodily processes are functions of the larger (meta) process scientists have named "the unconscious."

Since it is almost never consciously created and maintained, disease like digestion, is a creation of the unconscious. In order to achieve healing, it is necessary to establish a connection between the patient's waking consciousness and everything else in the universe; that is, the unconscious which is creating the disease. In his *Psychology and Alchemy* Dr. Jung observes that the concept of God may be validly substituted for the term 'unconscious.' Discourse with God is the province of the clergyman, but dialogue with the unconscious, he feels, is the valid concern of the doctor seeking to help his patient. His researches into alchemy led him to suggest that the image-making power of the human mind is the means by which the two are linked. The pictures you see on the backs of your closed eyelids are messages. They are trying to tell you something. In order to help his patients get the message, Dr. Jung devised the technique he calls active imagination.

> "Take the unconscious in one of its handiest forms,
> say a spontaneous fantasy ...concentrate on it, and
> observe its alterations. This fantasy is a real psychic
> process which is happening to you personally... If
> you recognize your own involvement you enter into
> the process with your own personal reactions, just as
> if you were one of the fantasy figures, or rather, as if
> the drama being enacted before your eyes were real."

The avowed purpose is to integrate the statements of the unconscious and to produce healing, or wholeness.

Sarah-Aphrodite healed her cancerous uterus by making pictures in her head. This case and a number of similar case histories in our files tend to bear out Jung's statement that it is "an undeniable fact that causal connections exist between the psyche and the body which point to their underlying unitary nature."

Like the pictures in your head, the symptoms in your body are messages. They are trying to tell you something. Physical disability and pain are means by which the unconscious psychic process combats external factors and conscious attitudes which impede progress toward its own goal. That goal is evolution. The battleground is the body. The symptoms increase in intensity until such time as the patient makes the required changes in his or her thought pattern. The method of active imagination of Jung offers a means for the resolution of the conflict between the patient's conscious mind and his unconscious psyche.

PSYCHIC HEALING MADE SIMPLE

1. Relax the body completely—in bed just before falling asleep is best.
2. Count backwards from five to zero, visualizing each number three times.
3. At the count of 0, you will see within the 0 a picture of the cause of the patient's difficulty—you will know it when you see it.
4. Erase the picture and substitute an image of your patient in perfect health. This can be found on the reverse side of the 0. It is not unusual for this to take place while dreaming.

If you choose to work during times when you will not immediately fall asleep, it is well to count back up from zero to five before resuming normal activities. Since the process involves no transfer of energy, your patient may be anywhere in the world. It is well to practice on your own minor illnesses and annoyances until you are convinced that it works.

In my own experience, during the course of a training session, I was given the intials of a woman in another city and asked to make a psychic diagnosis. In the center of my screen, I clearly saw an image of a right humerus (upper arm bone). There was an oblique line running through the shaft, separating an upper purple portion from a lower blue one. My diagnosis of an oblique fracture of the right humerus was correct. The picture which flashed in my head and the lady with the broken arm are connected because they both manifest at the same instant. In his idea of *synchronicity* Jung suggested that the flow of images which present themselves to our consciousness spontaneously (as dreams, visions, hallucinations, and guided imagery) and those that present themselve spontaneously through the five senses (empirical reality) are two aspects of a single phenomenon. The picture you make in your head is a hologram in the sense that it contains all the information necessary to reconstruct any aspect of its opposite pole (empirical reality) as it manifests at that same instant in time.

According to this concept, people can read each other's thoughts and send messages and pictures to each other by simultaneously concentrating on their inner images—the center of the 0. If they so command it, their inner screen will produce the same image or thought for each participant. In the case of picture or photograph transmission the sender concentrates on holding the image in his mind while the receiver commands his image-making process to reproduce it. Russian scientists classify these as bioinformational events, and claim they train operators as they would train athletes.

Using the technique described above, anyone can learn to be a healer. It is much easier than learning to walk on a tight rope. It is much easier even than learning to walk in the first place. It requires only that you devote yourself and practice 15 minutes a day.

On American TV an Israeli named Uri Geller bends a key using the force of his mind. In Leningrad, a Russian lady named Nelya Kulagina moves a cigarette across the table using the same energy source. In the United States, Olga Worral heals tumors by touching them. Down-to-earth, respectable people are coming back from the Philippines claiming to have been cured of far-advanced cancer by *psychic surgery.* The amount of data of this type being reported from institutions of unquestionable integrity demands that we reexamine our basic assumptions as to the nature of our physical world.

VI

We must face the mounting evidence for psychokinesis—mind affecting matter in space—even though it challenges the common sense tradition of 300 years. Psychokinesis, the application of mind over matter, is no more difficult than scratching an itch. I move the physical matter of my fingernail to a precise point in space. The mind controls the movement of matter. This power of mind extends outward to include inanimate matter like keys or cigarettes, and inward to our living cells, tissues, and organs. A new paradigm is being proposed by eminent members of the scientific community: the world is crystallized thought.

The practical implications of seeing mind and matter as a unity instead of as a duality are enormous. Reality, a unity, presents itself to us in two apparently opposite aspects—mind and matter. Current theory visualizes empirical reality as vibrating between my sensory impression ·of it, and my thoughts about it—the one creating the other. Not only is *my liver* not the same as it was at birth, it is not the same as it was the last time I thought about it. Matter is said to exist in four states, depending on its energy level or vibratory rate.

Depending on the rate of vibration, the element water manifests as solid ice, a liquid which can change its shape, and invisible gas—water vapor, or as a loose association of charged particles called plasma.

A thought in your head, the matter of your body, or the glasses on your face are vibratory energy tuned to different frequencies, just as what comes out of your radio depends on which frequency is selected. In one European lab they feel that if they had the proper tools they could plot the frequency combinations which create what we know as a house fly.

The nature and characteristics of this vibratory energy, were the subject of a Moscow meeting in 1972. The conference was arranged by Dr. Stanley Krippner, director of the Maimonides Hospital Dream Lab in Brooklyn, and Dr. E. Naumov, coordinator of research in the field of psychoenergetics and director of Moscow's Institute of Technical Parapsychology. The participants were Russian and American scientists with representatives from Canada, England, Austria, Italy, Czechoslovakia, Switzerland, Ireland, and the Federal German Republic—about 60 in all. The author participated in a section on practical applications in the field of healing.

Dr. Naumov noted that investigations in the field of psychic phenomena (psychoenergetics is the official Soviet term) have been actively pursued in the U.S.S.R. since 1919, interrupted only by World War II. Referring to Dr. Edgar Mitchell's successful transmission of mental images from the moon to earth during his Apollo flight, he made the following observations. "It is interesting to note that the last experiment carried out by Dr. Mitchell is very similar to the investigations performed by the pioneers of this work in our country. The existence of biologic communication (telepathy) has now been established. It is currently the object of serious scientific scrutiny in many countries throughout the world. This area of scientific research has greater import for humanity than the investigation of the cosmos itself. In the future space exploration human telepathic ability will be necessary and vital."

He offered the following definition for the Soviet researcher's term *psychoenergetics*, the equivalent of the American *psi phenomena:* "The field of investigation which studies sensitivity phenomena in living systems which are unexplained by the activity of the usual sense organs."

The researchers in Russia concern themselves with two main classes of phenomena: *ESP* (extrasensory perception) or *bioinformational* events characterized by exchange of energy which is predominately of a perceptual-sensory nature. This exchange takes place between living systems, and is exemplified by the works of Krippner and Mitchell.

Dr. Krippner had experimented with volunteers: the receiver went to sleep at the Dream Laboratory where his eye movements and brain waves were monitored. In another part of the city, the sender was given a photograph to study. The sender attempted to transmit the image into the dreams of the receiver by concentration. When the receiver indicated by rapid eye movements that he was dreaming, he was awakened and asked to describe his dream images. Next day he was presented with a packet of 100 photos, and asked to select the one used by the sender. In a statistically significant number of trials, the receiver included elements of the sender's image. The number of correct guesses identifying the test photos also exceeded that to be expected from random chance.

The Russian scientists reported successful experiments of their own with telepathic transmission of verbal and visual imagery over great distances. It was noted that the military of both countries are actively engaged in research in this area.

Psychokinesis (*PK*) or *bioenergetic* events are those processes in which the motor-kinetic aspect predominates. This phenomenon takes place as an exchange of energy between living and nonliving systems as well as between living systems. Examples of this type are seen in the phenomenon of psychic healing, or conversely, in mind-induced psychosomatic disease.

Professor Victor Adamenko of Moscow's Institute of Radio-Physics is interested in the phenomenon of psychokinesis as it manifests between living and nonliving systems. He has been training people to move objects up to 10 grams in weight without touching them. He introduced a young woman named Alla Vinogravada, who is also his wife, who explained that in order to perform PK, she must first work herself into a highly emotional state. Her blood pressure and heart rate rise

sharply and she becomes extremely agitated. She stated that
she was able to concentrate this accumulated energy first to
her fingertips, and then to the object she was trying to move. A
film was shown in which she moved cigar tubes, matchboxes,
wooden and metal squares, all by placing her hand about 3 - 6
inches away. The experiments lasted three minutes and were
terminated when her electrocardiogram showed signs of
cardiac strain. A school psychologist, she practices yoga to keep
in good physical health and limits her PK work so as not to
produce excessive physical and psychological strain.

Adamenko, a physicist who is also deeply interested in
acupuncture, then told how he studied Vinogravada's acupuncture points with the tobioscope, and instrument which
measures electrical resistance in the skin. Normal skin resistance, he stated, is around 500,000 ohms. Over the acupuncture
points the reading drops to 14,000 ohms. During the PK
sessions, rapid shifts in the electrical conductivity of these
points were noted. He also showed Kirlian photographs—a
cameraless electrical technique which captures on film a colorful aura of corona surrounding the body that changes with a
person's emotional, mental, or physical state—taken of Alla
Vinogravada in her ordinary state of mind and while she was
involved in PK. In the latter state, the flares were concentrated
at the fingertips and showed a change in color pattern from an
even blue green to splotchy and red.

The photographic results were interpreted as support for
Vinogravada's contention that she was able to convert psychologic energy into kinetic energy. The intensity of the electrostatic field induced at Vinogravada's fingertips varied, but
sometimes reached 100,000 volts. She could move an object
from as far away as two feet. She could slide 10 gram weights
(matchboxes) and cause 100 gram cylinders to roll away from
her outstretched fingers, working best when her hands were
dry and her confidence was high. Her ability seemed increased
during the evening and during the full moon. In conclusion,
Dr. Adamenko stated, "The data acquired in the course of
these experiments give us some idea as to how we may investigate the biological and electrical fields which surround the
body and the extent to which they may be controlled by
voluntary means."

Dr. V. M. Inyushin, a physicist at Kazakh University in the Soviet Union, postulated that the PK effect was analagous to that of a surface or object becoming electrically charged by lightening: "Psychokinesis represents the interaction of an object's electrostatic and electromagnetic fields with the fields of the human operator." He advanced the theory that a previously unrecognized state of matter, which he calls *bioplasma*, is associated with PK, acupuncture, and other so-called *paranormal* phenomena. This plasma state consists of a cloud of subatomic particles which is in dynamic equilibrium with the solids, liquids, and gases forming living tissue; perhaps even transforming itself into these other states from time to time, just as water becomes steam or ice. The highly ionized particles of the *biological plasma body* surround the living organism and penetrate its substance. He suggested that the acupuncture meridian system which carried bioplasmic energy is as important a component of the living body as the circulatory, lymphatic, and nervous systems. Currently, Dr. Inyushin is studying the voluntary control of internal states through yoga, brain wave biofeedback and other means.

I came back from the Moscow meetings with a great deal to think about. All this new information had to be integrated into my medical model and applied to making patients well. If mind and matter are not a duality, it is possible to construct a model wherein my mind can control my lung. Thought pattern shapes the flow of bioplasmic energy which lowers its vibratory rate and precipitates a lung. If a person thinks, "I'm an asthmatic and I have bad lungs," he usually has some mental picture which depicts a rotted lung, a stuffed breathing tube or something similar. William Tiller, professor of Materials Sciences at Stanford University, suggests that this thought pattern or mental picture is transmitted holographically and reproduces itself in matter. Flip Wilson, sums it up when he says, "What you see is what you get."

Our work with the modality called *sonopuncture* was stimulated by talks with other workers at the Moscow Conference. Of particular interest was the work with laser stimulation of the acupuncture system reported by Dr. Inyushin. In one experiment a student was able to work himself up into a rage reaction, raising his blood pressure, heart rate, and causing red flaring on Kirlian photos of his extremities. Low intensity laser light was then directed to the acupuncture points in the hand. This maneuver reversed the physiologic changes and prevented him from reproducing the bodily changes associated with anger. Preliminary work with lasers at Kazakh University Medical Center shows reversal of malignant bone tumors and restitution of normal tissue. It was the feeling of Dr. Inyushin that stimulation of the acupuncture meridian system by sound might be as effective as light stimulation. He suggested we try it and evaluate its efficacy.

Acupuncture consists of conscious rebalancing of the primal cosmic forces in the patient. The meridians are divided into yin, which are localized in the front and interior part of the body, and yang, which run along the back and are found on the external body surface. The former are related to maintenance functions such as breathing, digestion, and metabolism. Yang is the energy of defense. Sites of application of energy are determined by the time of day, time of year, and by the pulses according to a relatively easy to learn blueprint. (Life-size charts which outline and describe the locations of the channels are readily available at book stores.) During the fall and afternoon, we follow the procedure known as yin tonification. In cases where the patient is depressed and debilitated we are advised to tonify (boost) the yang. Workers at other clinics are making progress in the control of heroin withdrawal by means of this method of energy manipulation. One of our patients reported the subjective effects of yin tonification as equivalent to those achieved after several hours of Kundalini Yoga. The full effects of treatment take 24 hours to manifest, while residual effects have been noted to last a week or longer. One consistent effect of successful treatment is a profound sense of subjective physical and mental well-being.

Our preliminary study at Headlands using high frequency sound indicates about 80% effectiveness in a randomly selected sample of 100 general practice problems. Massage, heat, and directed attention can also regulate the energy flow. Manipulating the energy patterns changes the state of the internal tissue of organs fed by the meridian and healing can be achieved.

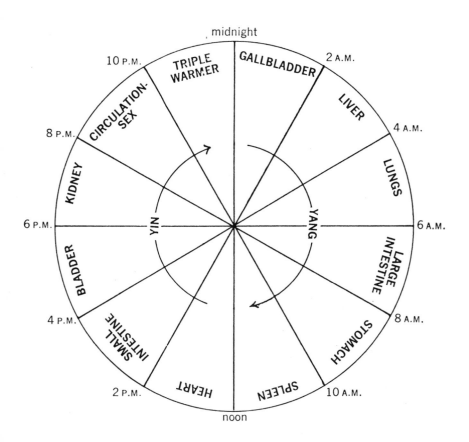

LAW OF ACUPUNCTURE (Noon-Midnight)
Certain times of the day are best for treatment of specific organs.
Yin and Yang organs respond best at the time of day they are most
active. Treating one organ will also affect the organ opposite it.

One particularly impressive case involved the use of sono-puncture anesthesia. An 11-year-old boy had a bike accident which resulted in the impaction of a twig the size of a knitting needle into his thigh. The end had disappeared and was deep in the muscle. Removal under general anesthesia in an operating room is the usual approach. Since he was a regular patient, he was familiar with the sonopuncture technique. While we applied sound to the proper acupuncture point for anesthesia the patient was able to push the inside end of the twig until it protruded from the skin and permitted the application of a hemostat to grab the exposed end. Dr. Wexler, of our staff, then leaned back on his heels and yanked the foreign body out of the muscle. The patient experienced no pain during or after the procedure. There was no sign of trauma to the leg other than the entrance wound. He resumed his normal activities immediately afterward and suffered none of the aftereffects that might be expected from this type of wound.

The boy is still under our care. He is on a bimonthly treatment program to prevent recurrent asthmatic attacks which have plagued him most of his life. In the course of his first visit, he was able to abort an acute asthmatic episode by picturing a vacuum cleaner "zooping out his breathing tubes." He had no difficulty accepting the ritual. He had never read Descartes; he trusted us completely, and he hates hospitals.

VII

Joe works at the general store. He is of above average intelligence. "Can you tell me what to do to get my ear unstuffed?" He blew his nose last night and apparently forced some mucus into his eustachian tube.

Upon being advised that it is necessary to examine the eardrum in order to determine the best treatment, he frowns. "Isn't there something simple I can do which will unclog my tube?"

"Can you make pictures in your head?"

"You mean you want me to make a picture of my eustachian tube opening?"

"Yeah."

"Thanks a lot." He turns back to the cash register, muttering under his breath.

Television advertising, unlike Joe, recognizes the power of the image. In one example a construction worker is shown leaving work because of a headache and some fever. By the time he gets home he is coughing and sweating, and later confined to bed— all the symptoms of pneumonia. After taking two of the advertised pills, he's shown back at work, fresh as a daisy and raring to go! A more skillful approach represents the victim's clogged sinuses in the form of a superimposed sink drain replacing his nose. Popping the prescribed pill causes the drain to open, emptying the stuffed sinus/sink, which then changes into a happy smile.

The next step in our investigation at the Headlands Healing Service was boosted by a retired analyst who had espoused the theory exemplified by the Silva Mind Control School. This school, and many others like it, claim to be able to teach an average individual with average intelligence effective mind control in a short period of time—as little as 48 hours. Their goals are essentially the same: "increased intelligence, an improved memory, heightening of extrasensory perceptive abilities, more incisive and intuitive problem-solving powers, and better control of human emotions and bodily functions. The movement also has encountered controversy, however, because some of its schools also purport to enable people to correct physical conditions ranging from migraine headaches to terminal cancer. Insomnia, drug and alcohol addiction, overeating, and cigarette smoking are just a few of the undesirable behavioral manifestations which mind control also can correct, its advocates say." [11]

Our teacher was known around the clinic as "Murray-Mind-Control." He just appeared one day and said he would like us to examine the technique in our clinical setting. A veteran of 25 years as a practicing psychotherapist, he announced, "I'm going to teach your guys how to do it. I will make psychics out of all of you in ten days...Maybe we can cut it to four. You'll do psychic diagnosis, telepathy...you'll do it all." He did it in four days.

Using a simple hypnotic technique, he taught 25 of the local citizenry, selected at random, to enhance and manipulate their spontaneous mental images. Creating a vivid picture of healing resulted in healing on the somatic level. The patient was asked to visualize his pathology, and create an image of healing. A patient with glaucoma was able to reduce her intraocular pressure to normal by picturing fluid running out of her eyeballs through a spigot. Merely visualizing the tonometry instrument registering the desired pressure was effective. Her opthalmologic consultant who was monitoring her status felt that we had proved nothing because "she was able to reduce her pressure from time to time by an act of will." A second patient with glaucoma was able to reduce the pressure in one eye consistently. She decided she would fare better with the help of a Reichian analyst.

Skin problems responded well: in two cases, poison oak dermatitis resolved completely within 30 minutes after the initiation of therapy. Children responded particularly well, probably because they have no preconceptions and are willing to entertain the possibility of immediate cure. We instituted a training program in the town which would help people sharpen their ability to visualize. It is interesting to note that while over a hundred people received the training, very few used the technique in the face of ordinary common illnesses. Word got around that the clinic was engaged in weird mystical activities and was to be avoided.

What we were actually trying to do was show *the way* in which an individual can maintain himself in perfect health and, if necessary, heal himself. While accepted by the people in theory, they rejected it in returning to the rituals they had been educated to believe in. In accepting the old, familiar mode of healing, they were seeking to repress symptoms rather than remove themselves from an ego-centered state and examine the actual cause by contacting the unconscious. However we elect to contact the unconscious domain (meditation is most common), the energy must flow from it in the form of a visual image. The conscious domain commands that a picture be created which depicts the energy or message of the symptom.

Sound ridiculous? Consider the work of Carl Simonton, M.D. Depressed because so many of his cancer patients were dying in spite of X-radiation of the tumors, he utilized visual imagery in his treatment program. One case involved a B-52 navigator with a far-advanced malignancy of the throat. It had reached the size of a peach and was occluding the openings to the lungs and stomach. There was evidence of spread. Faced with certain death, the patient agreed to try the technique. He was taught to enter the alpha state by means of complete body relaxation. In this state, he visualized his white blood cells in the form of cowboys on horseback. The defenders were then seen attacking and destroying the cancer cells. The procedure was repeated three times daily for 15 minutes. Over a period of seven weeks the tumor receded in size and finally disappeared, leaving a normal throat mucosa. At the end of this time, he was taken back to the operating room, where biopsy specimens revealed only normal tissue.

In September of 1973, Dr. Simonton reported success in 128 cases using the combination of X-ray and visual imagery. The degree of success was proportional to the cooperative effort of the patient. Dr. Simonton's position as a director of the prestigious American Cancer Society gives additional credence to his claims.

Dr. Simonton's evolution paralleled my own and is worth noting. At a symposium sponsored by the Academy of Parapsychology and Medicine in 1972, he said, "While the young physician is under all the pressures of current concepts and limitations both from the system itself and the people who teach him, at the same time he feels a tremendous responsibility to make right decisions. He *must* always be right, for fear that in being wrong he may endanger someone's health or life. This fear causes him to accept the medical teachings that are given to him. He hesitates to think much on his own for fear his wrong thinking may cause further ill health or ultimately death on the part of a patient. This feeling is largely generalized in our thinking, and during these focal years we have a tendency to be very close-minded because of this tremendous, overwhelming fear."

Later he was influenced by a prominent immunotherapist who had a remarkable success in the treatment of terminal leukemic patients. "He indeed went ahead and developed this (treatment) and achieved a 50% remission rate...other investigators immediately attempted to reproduce these results. But there is one essential difference between the initial investigator's approach and that of those attempting to reproduce his work, and that is that the idea was his idea to begin with—an idea about which he was very enthusiastic—a quality which is lacking in the approach of subsequent investigators."

Dr. Simonton explained that "The initial investigator had taken more pains to explain to the patients and their families the basic mechanisms and the expected results; he had taken a very much more intensified approach. The subsequent experiments by other investigators showed approximately one-half as good results as his initial work had shown. After these less favorable reports were published, subsequent investigators were even more skeptical of the possible good of such forms of therapy, and further investigations showed a corresponding decrease in response of the patients treated."

He then took up the examination of the extensive cancer cases that have unexplained "good results." After only a short time, "it became very clear to me that there was one strong factor that seemed to run through each history...(the patient's) attitude toward the disease and his basic attitude toward life... It then behooved me to learn how to teach attitude— the will to live, or whatever you want to call it—to my patients." Dr. Simonton then began a search for a methodology to change attitude; he analyzed the methods of successful salesmen and eventually discovered biofeedback. Finally, following completion of a mind control course, he felt confident that he had learned enough about the power of the mind to teach attitude to his patients.

"The following Monday I started the process with my first patient. In addition to the medical treatment, I explained what my thinking was, I told him how, through mutual imagery, we were going to attempt to affect his disease. He was a 61-year-old gentleman with very extensive throat cancer. He had lost a great deal of weight, could barely swallow his own saliva, and could eat no food. After explaining his disease and the way radiation worked, I had him relax three times a day, mentally picture his disease, his treatment, and the way his body was interacting with the treatment and the disease, so that he could better understand his disease and cooperate with what was going on. The results were truly amazing... That patient is now a year and a half post-treatment, with no evidence of cancer in his throat. He also had arthritis, and he used the same basic mental process and eliminated that."

The administrative staff of the USAF Medical Center was receptive to his ideas and he was allowed to develop his revolutionary healing technique. "The first fifty patients we treated at Travis were divided into attitude groups, going from double negative to double positive. Five members of the department graded these patients individually, and then we averaged the results. Next, we classified the results from poor to excellent. We found a direct line of correlation between poor attitudes and poor responses, with good attitudes correspondingly showing good responses. One exciting point here is that only four out of fifty patients had a poor response, and this includes all patients that came through the door for treatment, including very intensive disease. Out of the fifty, thirty-seven (or 74%) had either good or excellent responses; and 12% had excellent response. ...eight of the twelve had less than a 50% chance for cure, and four of the twelve had better than a 50% chance for cure." [12]

Supporting these observations is a study done by a group of physicians and psychologists at the New Orleans Veterans Hospital. Twenty-one patients with high blood pressure, ranging in age from 23 to 65, participated. Nine patients received standard drug treatment and six received no medication. The remaining six received no treatment at all and served as controls. The first two groups were hypnotized and told to relax internal organs including heart and arteries. The typical patient, whether on drugs or not, was able to reduce blood pressure to within normal limits by the second or third session. The mental image of relaxed organs were reproduced on the physical level—psychokinesis: a plausible explanation for the positive results.

An American pole-vaulting champion says that he pictures himself clearing the desired height about 100 times. The actual jump is then one more repetition of the event. Evel Knievel can do things on a motorcycle which no other human has been able to do. In a recent television interview he described his technique for jumping his cycle over 17 trucks: "I get that motorcycle up there, and I just *see* it flying over all those trucks, and landing on the other side."

What about all those people who visualize what they want and don't get it? Do they have subconscious wishes and urges which run contrary to professed desires and motivations?

We can probe for the answers to some of these difficult questions by applying the scientific method. This requires that we examine the observed facts and data with an open mind. A mountain of observations and data is now presenting itself which refuses to fit into the Cartesian's cosmologic mold. For three hundred years we have said these things didn't *really* happen, attacking the reporters of this work as mystics and cranks.

Descarte's theory like Newtonian physics, was a casualty of the atomic bomb. Matter, the irreducible reality, was shown to be a form of energy. Both world views fell victim to the fact that a significant amount of empirical data, like psychokinesis, fails to conform to their models. By refusing to reexamine their basic premise in the light of contradictory evidence, Cartesian scientists run the risk of themselves falling into the trap of cultism. The Cartesians should reconsider the thoughts of philosopher Bertrand Russell first published in 1927: "For aught we know an atom may consist entirely of the radiations which come out of it. It is useless to argue that radiations cannot come out of nothing... The idea that there is a little lump there, which *is* the electron or proton, is an illegitimate intrusion of commonsense notions derived from touch... Matter is a convenient formula for describing what happens where it isn't." [13]

Our concept of reality is created by our need to explain catabolic forces. These impersonal, superhman forces manifest as earthquakes, floods, and fires. In society we encounter them in the form of war, crime, famine, and social disintegration. On the personal level their equivalent is disease, mental anguish, and most recently, demonic possessions. The disasters that periodically befall humanity, individually and collectively, are said to be caused by the activity of matter. These lumps and aggregations of matter, this irreducible ultimate reality, are supposed to exist independently of perceiving consciousness—if a tree falls in the forest, it makes a noise whether or not anyone hears it. This matter, what the philosopher Alan

Watts calls *stuff*, [14] is what Cartesian scientists have been accepting uncritically for over 300 years.

The Cartesian splitting of thought and substance into polar opposites presumes their unity on a higher level. This higher unity has the power to initiate a wave of cosmic energy causing man's society to disintegrate and his emotions to run riot. Consider the quasar reaching earth on Black Tuesday; most religious texts speak of the periodic flood which washes away civilization and almost all its inhabitants.

In addition to the catabolic aspect, this unification of opposites (God or whatever) has an anabolic or constructive aspect. Since time immemorial humans have either built arks to survive the flood, wandered 40 years in wilderness, or communed with this omniscient unity on mountain tops in order to turn off an atrocious empirical reality. Most of the adaptations to the destructive nature of the unity, are described as having been derived from visions: Buddha's encounter under the Bo tree with the Lord of Death, or Christ's temptation by the Devil on the mountain. Applying the Russian model of bioplasmic energy, we might say that the mental image which appears to consciousness during meditative (alpha-theta) states flashes holographically the direction and nature of the prevailing energy burst in the cosmos.

An immediate application of this thesis would be to take 15 minutes a day to get a cosmic weather report, so to speak. Human consciousness, specifically the rational function, has the power to initiate vibrations in the bioplasma. When the thinker (oscillator) is at rest, it vibrates in the alpha range (about 10 cycles/second)—this is the basic vibratory rate of the field of planet earth. Bioplasmic energy enters the body, traverses the twelve acupuncture meridians where it precipitates the organs in a steady state of vibration between matter and energy. If we do nothing, Chinese authors tell us, cosmic energy rebalances of its own accord and restores harmony.

> Sitting quietly,
>> doing nothing,
>>> the grass grows green and spring comes.

The energy charge you feel in your gut, chest, or wherever, might have originated in, a quasar or in an exploding star system which no longer exists. You may blame your bed companion or anyone else, but if you consider you will observe that the energy grabs you from outside or inside. You then formulate a *reason* for feeling the energy: "I was grouchy," "you started it," "I'm depressed," etc. The alchemical approach would be to seal the energy hermetically, do not run it off in worries, arguments, or general thrashing about, as this route generally results in tissue destruction and premature aging.

Do not give the feeling any name except energy, concentrate on making your breath regular and even. Observe the effect this has on the energy. Make a simple mental picture of the energy, and visualize it flowing up the front and down the back of your body. Any pattern of the flow which *feels* right works. Consider physical symptoms to be blockages of free flow of the energy. While giving your full attention to breathing regularly and circulating the energy, check each part of your body for obstructions to the flow. While you are doing this, expect to see a visual image in your head which represents total health. You'll know it when you see it, it will affect you like the flag affects the patriot. The *charge* you feel is the energy of the *lousy mood* or of the *ache.* Its polarity has been reversed; it shows its benign instead of its destructive face; this face, manifesting as healing.

VIII

It is suggested that the world is crystallized thought. By that we mean that your mental image of empirical reality may possibly be creating that reality. If this is true, then the advice to stop thinking and remain quiet during periods of stress may well be considered. During this period of rest for the left-sided thinker, the right-sided visual-image can be used to program a state of complete healing.

If we adopt the reality model of modern physics and accept the premise that everything is made of the same basis material, atoms, we must also presume that there is no stomach nor ulcer. An excellent example of this idea would be the way in which we select groupings of stars and call them constellations. Likewise, a grouping of atoms in particular circumstances has been labeled *stomach*. There is only a constant flux of atomic energy which by changing its pattern creates that which we call stomach, and recreates it anew from instant to instant.

We can use the model of a biocomputer with over 10 billion terminals which constitutes the human brain. (The largest man-made computers have 100,000 terminals.) The function of this computer is to project reality into what we

call time and space. This includes the reality of the physical
body as well as that of the environment. By programming the
biocomputer we create our total physical reality. There is
a great deal of scientific evidence accumulating to support this
thesis. There is nothing *out there* independent of our perception of it. Mental imagery seems to play the role of a programming punch card to this computer. This therapeutic approach
requires getting the computer into a state where it will accept
reprogramming—the alpha state.

Dr. Jeffery J. Smith of Stanford University has examined
areas of parapsychology and uses the alpha state of meditation
to attempt to understand reality. At Stanford, Dr. Smith had
an opportunity to observe and discuss with physicists from
Stanford Research Institute, the remarkable feats of Uri
Geller. "Do you always know when the powers will manifest
themselves?" I asked. "No," he answered, "Sometimes they
come quite unexpectedly." At which point the fork poised in
his hand simply buckled. A moment later he added,
"Sometimes they dont't just bend; they break." At which point
the untouched spoon beside him simply broke.

"...if phenomena such as the spoon break are genuine,
they call for a radical revision of both our current conception
of reality and our current conception of science."

"For some time the basic scientific conception of reality
has been that the physical is primary, and that life is a
secondary and mind a tertiary derivative. This conception
may be overt or covert, bald or sophisticated, blunt or attenu-
ated. But it is there, in the physical, social, and humanistic
sciences. This focus on the physical has been immensely
productive, but has generated problems that threaten to
destory us..."

"Consider once again the broken spoon. This was apparently both a mental and a physical event. Note the way the
bending of the fork and breaking of the spoon seemed to enter
into the conversation. It was as though consciousness and
meaning were at work in the metal itself. Suppose they were
poltergeist phenomena, springing from some unfathomed part
of Uri's unconscious. Then we must deepen and enlarge our
notion of the unconscious, for the phenomena took place in

what has been marked off as the domain of physics. But can we stop there? Shall we patch things up by saying that mind seems to radiate a little further than we had thought? Or shall we postulate a mind-energy, dimension or field of a more cosmic nature?" [15]

Drs. Alyce and Elmer Green of the Menninger Clinic refer to the *field of mind* theory. We could postulate that the known field of electromagnetic energy surrounding and penetrating our planet represents the field of mind vibrating within a given range of frequencies. The color red has a particular rate of vibration within the frequency band representing the phenomenon of light. Color frequency range could now be conceived as lying within the field of mind which could be thought of as the electromagnetic spectrum extended at each end to infinity.

In the case of visual light, human consciousness perceives differing wave lengths as totally different phenomena—colors. The range of frequencies perceivable by our five sensory receptors as external reality makes up the world of matter. It is a tiny portion of the total known electromagnetic spectrum. It is an infinitesimal speck in the band of infinitely possible numbers of vibratory rates. Within this band lies the narrower frequency range which our consciousness perceives as the physical (somatic) body. Human awareness is said to register higher vibratory rates as thought or imagery, and changing a mental image, is able to transform the somatic experience and cure the disease. The Greens conclude: "The normally involuntary, unconscious, sections of one's self can be induced to behave in ways that are consciously chosen by visualizing what is wanted, asking the being (body, mind, brain, unconscious, or whatever) to do it, and then detaching oneself from the results. A symbolic way of putting it is to say that the cortex plants the impulse in the subcortex and then allows nature to take its course without interference."

If, as is claimed by Eastern cosmologies, mind, matter and energy are all the same—a unity—we would expect each member of the trinity to transform into either of the other aspects, like in a hologram where the image contains all the information necessary to reconstruct the object (a hologram is a three-dimensional image projected in space by a laser beam of congruent light).

Kirlian, or high-voltage, photography is a method of producing an image of energy fields or auras that surround the bodies of living things using electricity in place of a light source. The process has many fascinating implications and could well be an important diagnostic tool for the future.

In the late 19th century, the Austrian-born electrician and inventor, Nikola Tesla, gave a public demonstration of electricity being used to illuminate and make visible the energy field. By saturating himself with electricity he was able to give off a glow which he described as "streams of light" originating from his body. The process has been experimented with and refined by scientists in the United States and Russia, obtaining its name, Kirlian, from a Russian inventor who was instrumental in its development.

The photographs are made on color or black and white film, in the absence of light, as follows:
1. The fingers are placed on unexposed film between two conductor plates, preferably copper.
2. A potential electrical difference is created between the plates of 25,000 volts for 4-8 seconds.
3. The film is developed in the usual manner.
4. The photographs are examined and the implications are considered.

The cameraless electrical technique purportedly captures on film a colorful aura or corona surrounding the body that changes with a person's emotional, mental, or physical state, thereby giving rise to speculation that it might become as significant a tool for medicine as EEGs, ECGs, or X-rays. Many of its American investigators, however, seem equally enthusiastic about its potential for unraveling mysteries surrounding acupuncture, psychic phenomena such as extrasensory perception and psychokinesis, and healing by the mystics' method of "laying on of hands." The process, they add, might confirm the existence of long suspected but as yet unknown energy forces in the body—perhaps representing *prana* described by Yoga philosophy thousands of years ago, Wilhelm Reich's orgones, or bioplasma, a name coined by the

Soviets. Both the medical and parapsychological applications have been gaining widespread coverage, ranging from articles in *Psychic Magazine* to a front-page news story for laymen in the *Wall Street Journal* and an 11-page technical report in a recent issue of the *Journal of Applied Physics.*

In an experiment carried out by UCLA's Dr. Thelma Moss, marijuana smoking changes a subject's fingertip coronas from skimpy partial halos to large luminous bursts of pink and crimson. Dr. Moss finds that relaxation induced by drugs usually results in more brilliant coronas.

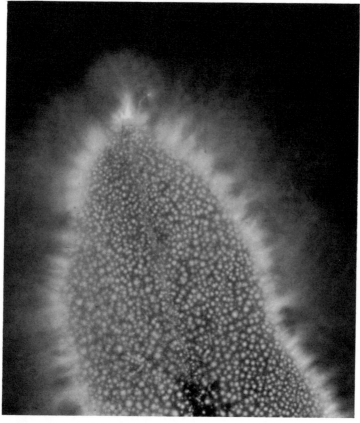

This is a Kirlian Photograph of a leaf.

Dr. Moss is also using Kirlian photography to investigate possible mechanisms entailed in acupuncture. She notes that the Chinese have traditionally considered acupuncture meridians as energy channels in the body. In one of her experiments, needles were placed in the knee of a patient with chronic pain in the ball of the foot. The treatment site conformed to a meridian said by the Chinese to influence the foot. Kirlian images of the patient's foot before and after therapy appeared to show a definite energy change, says Dr. Moss.

Another of her investigations concerns hypothetical energy transfers brought about by faith healing. In a three-month experiment performed on 12 dialysis patients, a healer placed his hands on their back in the kidney region for 20 minutes each day. Fingertip photography taken of the healer showed that a rosy pink aura present before the "treatments" was absent afterwards. In contrast, pink was also nonexistent in the fingertip auras of patients before therapy but appeared prominentaly after it. With one exception, these effects were not obtained when nonhealers performed the laying on of hands. None of the patients were cured, although they sometimes showed some symptomatic improvement and often said they felt better and had experienced sensations of intense heat or tingling during the treatments. Dr. Moss considers the results interesting but inconclusive.

Within the past three years, an increasing number of American scientists have been expressing active interest in (this) eerie photographic technique that the Russians have been quietly working on for more than three decades. As matters stand now, the research has all the ingredients of a first-rate suspense yarn. It is laying the groundwork for a valuable new diagnostic system that may, for example, detect illnesses such as flu even before symptoms appear? Or is it simply a new form of pseudoscientific dabbling in the supernatural? [16]

During the past few years a story of remarkable occurrence has come to the attention of the medical profession. It concerns a Kirlian photograph taken of a leaf with a portion cut off and removed. On the print the cut line appears but the image and corona of the missing piece are also apparent. A

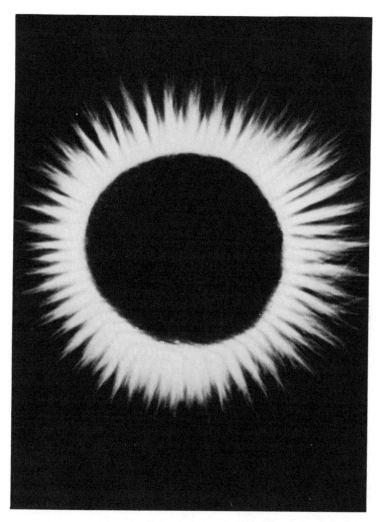

This photograph was made without a camera. The subject placed his fingers on unexposed film between two conductor plates, across which a difference of potential of 25,000 volts was created for four to eight seconds. The resulting images, called Kirlian photographs after their Russian inventor, show the aura emanating from the body. Some scientists who have studied auras believe that the electrical impulses which cause them are a function of emotional change.

great deal of time has been spent in the United States attempting to duplicate the achievement. All major controlled research attempts to replicate the effect have been unsuccessful; some individuals claim degrees of success but data concerning the experiments has not been corroborated.

More importantly and even more astounding was the recent success achieved by J. Hickman in experiments conducted with Uri Geller. In reporting the "formation of luminous images by conscious mental effort" during the making of Kirlian photographs, H. S. Dakin warns that they occur "so rarely, if at all, that for most practical purposes it may be considered as impossible."

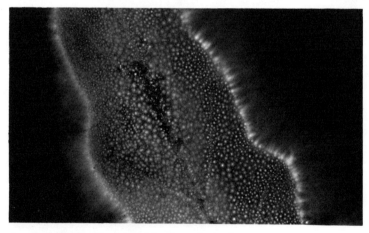

Another Kirlian Photographic view of a leaf.

A possible example of one of these rare instances is shown in high-voltage prints made in recent (December, 1973) experiments conducted by J. Hickman with U. Geller, a remarkable person already well-known for confounding physicists and psychologists with displays of apparent mental-physical energy interactions, causing metal objects to bend and break, and magnetic field-strength meters to show noticeable deflections accompanying intense concentration and muscle tension.

These photographs and others which should appear in a forthcoming report by J. Hickman were made in a series of experiments witnessed by J. Mayo, H. S. Dakin, W. Westerbeke, and S. Kenny, using a prototype model of the timer-controlled high-voltage supply...under conditions which offered little opportunity for using trickery to produce the results. The subject (Mr. Geller) had had no previous contact with the apparatus used in the experiments.

In each of the two examples shown, the subject announced that he together with the group of experimenters would concentrate intensely on a particular geometric form (first a circle, then a triangle) and try to project it by mental energy onto the film, under or near his fingerprint, at the same time as the high-voltage exposure. The circular image of the fingertip alone, with corona streamers radiating outward (as in the normal or control fingerprint exposures) is all that one would expect to see, unless other physical objects were present on the film. [17]

Exactly what is it that Kirlian photographs show? Where does the energy shown in the photographs emanate? Douglas Dean, former head of the Parapsychological Association, makes an interesting case for Kirlian photography being capable of demonstrating the healing power of a faith healer. "Four sets of photographs out of four show greatly increased flares when the suggestion to think of healing had been given...tentatively we can assume that the act of healing seems to produce increased flaring. [18]

IX

TO THE PHYSICIAN

Any idea or system which is not in accord with the pre-conceptions of 17th century scientific materialism is arbitrarily relegated to the status of cultism or, even worse, occultism. We seem to have forgotten that scientific materialism, as represented by Descartes, is merely a hypothesis concerning reality which demoted God and elevated matter to the status of ultimate reality. Empirical reality, the world, was not created by an old man with a gray beard in seven days. It was created, the theory says, by the blind forces of nature over a period of several billion years. These forces represent the part of our living experience which we accept as given. The vast majority of humans believe today that natural forces which we know as electromagnetism, gravity, inertia, etc., are created and controlled by some superterrestial mind, a preexisting consciousness which manipulates cosmic energy in an autocratic and sometimes capricious manner. My mind inhabits my body at the whim and pleasure of the landlord—God. The Cartesians promised we could make our survival in the realm of matter less tenuous by adopting their particular religious belief. The primal trinity, they say, consists of mind, matter, and energy.

The body and the world it lives in are composed of matter. Over and against this, we have a mind which inhabits the former in order to deal with the latter. René Descartes' idea that mind and matter are two separate things became axiomatic in what Arthur Koestler, a prominent American writer, calls "the Cartesian Catastrophe." Descartes' theory "stated that the world was composed of three elements formed from primitive matter. The first element...consisted of very subtle minute matter capable of moving at enormous speeds and of filling in the small spaces surrounding the other two denser forms of matter. The second element consisted of spherical particles formed from rotation of the original primitive matter. These spheres...moved in larger vortices at high speeds and could transmit pressure instantaneously. The third element was coarser and slower...(an) important aspect of Descartes' worldview was his belief in God's initial and continued action in the universe. God initially created matter in motion and set the vortices rotating. His continued recreation of the world from instant to instant guaranteed his presence in the creation..."

Newtonian physics tells us *how* energy affects *matter* in *space*. The *law of gravity* concept is an excellent example of the limitations of the Cartesian model. The mind of Sir Isaac Newton was in a body which was seated under an apple tree. An apple from the tree fell and struck the head of the body. Sir Isaac's mind then experienced a thought which goes something like, "Ahhh! Small clumps of matter are pulled toward large clumps of matter." This concept is known as the *law of mass attraction*. The preexistent, autonomous, blind force of nature which pulls smaller bodies in space toward larger bodies causing them to *fall* became known as the force of gravity.

A five-year-old child might respond to this information by asking, "Why did the apple fall?" The *law of gravity* tells us nothing about *why* the apple hit Sir Isaac on the head. It describes the event, the force acting in time, and gives it a name, explaining nothing. Our five-year-old innocent might have difficulty comprehending how this new, meaningless word answers his simple question. I must confess that I have the same difficulty. The idea that gravity is a manifestation of the workings of a rational cosmic mind is dismissed by the Cartesians as religious poppycock. The concept of Plato that the world is a concretized idea, of Buddha and Christ that empirical reality is merely an illusory projection of an ultimate inner reality, your own consciousness, is relegated by our Cartesian colleagues to the realm of metaphysical nonsense. It wasn't God who threw the apple at Newton's head, nor was it the *power of Newton's mind;* it was *gravity* they say.

Our modern period of Cartesian materialism may be considered a second Dark Age. We consider ourselves intellectually superior to the Chinese who invented paper and the Indian who developed and perfected the corn plant. We persist in embracing a medical model based on the assumption that matter exists continuously in space. We do this in the face of all evidence to the contrary, and in spite of the fact that 80% of patients' complaints are unresponsive to our therapeutics. Our consciousness took a quantum leap when we finally accepted the heresy that the world is round. Constantly exposed to varying concepts regarding the nature of reality, our consciousness usually selects the one that seems best for it, and adopts that view.

Medical theory, based on the Cartesian model, tells us that germs or other noxious agents come from *out there,* invade our bodies and make us sick. Modern physics tells us that our bodies are *open fields*—we are continuous with the cosmos and with each other. This is in direct contradiction to the Cartesian assumption that my physical being ends at my skin. It is obvious that what I think affects you and what you think affects the person sitting next to you. If someone who is extremely agitated enters a room we are aware of his state by its effect on our own composure—we can feel his presence. When any one of us exists in peace and seems contented, others are soothed by our presence; the state is contagious. It is possible to radiate peace or its opposite. By changing its demeanor from wrathful to peaceful the mind alters its vibratory rate in such a manner as to change the nature of its experience in the world of matter. When one is in a good mood, everything seems to go well, and the body functions at maximal efficiency. If we are angry or frustrated, everything seems to go wrong; the previously tranquil body begins to produce "gacid indigestion" and other annoying symptoms. If we merely stop thinking, everything becomes peaceful and the symptoms abate. One's thoughts may be creating one's physical reality. It is possible, dear reader, that we are making the whole thing up.

This, too, too solid flesh is an illusion. It is composed of subatomic particles which vibrate between states of existence and nonexistence. After three centuries of meticulous examination, modern physics declares that empirical reality (the world *out there*) is a figment of the imagination.

Man in the last quarter of the 20th century is experiencing a sudden increase, a quantum jump, in consciousness. The fact that we learned more about the planet Mercury yesterday than in the past 35,000 years illustrates the apocalyptic expansion rate of our consciousness. By a circumglobal television network we are in communication with all parts of our own planet; we have extended our senses to probe other members of our galaxy. Teilhard de Chardin describes this phenomenon as the extension of consciousness of the *noosphere*—the mantle of thought or ideas which engage humanity. Noosphere and *Field of Mind* are products of the same mental structure, as their obvious similarities indicate. Teilhard postulates consciousness itself as the primal preexisting cause of everything. The source of this preexisting consciousness is unknowable. Jung thinks it arose from the unconscious, the unknown. Both agree that it is evolving, shaping matter within the framework of the space-time continuum.

In the beginning, writes Teilhard, there was space. Suspended in infinite space is the total quantum of consciousness and of matter which constitutes our cosmos. It is dispersed into tiny hydrogen particles, equal parts of matter and consciousness, two sides of a single entity. Vast swirling clouds of consciousness-matter compress into complex atoms, compress further into molecules, compounds, mineral stones, and finally into the planet earth, the geosphere. This tendency to compression leads to more complex matter arrangements, higher levels of consciousness, until at the level of the nucleo-proteins, life—the cell—appears.

The spark of consciousness in the hydrogen atom has made a great leap. Enclosing itself in a membrane, it now manifests an inside and an outside, self and not self, the point within the circle. Immensely amplified, consciousness now directs an equally complexified matter toward positive and away from negative stimuli, it has become polarized. The primal drive toward complexification of matter and amplification of consciousness continues, first in the body—multicellular organisms showing more and more complex structures and manifesting a higher state of consciousness constitute the biosphere—the mantle of life on the surface of the earth. Consciousness then localizes at the front end where it devises a brain. As brain matter complexifies, consciousness-light amplifies. With the advent of Homo sapiens (the one who knows), another cataclysmic change occurs. Physical evolution gives way to the evolution of ideas in the realm of pure mind.

It is this force of evolution which has carried humanity out of the caves and into modern civilization. Urban civilized man, like his Cro-Magnon counterpart, begins life as a fertilized egg. Something causes that single cell to grow a head, arms, and legs, and to adopt the physical body characteristics of Homo sapiens. The configuration of the DNA molecules in the genes causes the raw stuff of life, protoplasm, to assume a shape conforming to the genetic code. Again, Cartesian science tells us how but offers no explanation of why a fertilized egg becomes a human being. If it seems unreasonable to propose that human beings are a device by which the fertilized egg reproduces itself, it is eminently reasonable to propose that human beings are a means by which consciousness reproduces and improves itself.

In the course of the journey from egg to newborn, the developing ovum replays the scenario of the evolution of physical form on the planet; from single cell to reptile, fish amphibian, and finally, after nine months, assuming the shape of a water-dwelling mammal, it gets its nourishment through a stalk (umbilical cord), attached by a root system to the maternal soil. At term, the human fetus is as much a plant as it is a person. At this point a catastrophe occurs. The life support system is ripped out by the roots, the water disappears, and life is cast out onto dry land. Any creature which does not adapt to this radical environmental change by a physical metamorphosis does not survive. Lungs must inflate, holes in the heart must close, and the blood is rerouted so that it can extract life-giving oxygen from air instead of from water. The process which the obstetrician calls birth is the death of the intrauterine plant mammal. The evolutionary process does not stop at this point.

At the period we call pubescence, the body changes again. The ovum develops secondary sex characteristics and perpares to reproduce. These spontaneous bodily changes impose themselves upon our consciousness. The child awakes one day to find he is somebody else. Insofar as the individual attempts to remain the same as he was before the onset of the physical metamorphosis, he adopts a thought pattern which is disharmonic with the flow of the evolutionary force. This flow of evolution never stops. We are always turning into somebody else, physically as well as mentally. My 12-year-old daughter, as her body was changing asked, "How come I suddenly get bored with all the things I loved to do when I was young?" This change in interest is a change in thought pattern, another facet of the spontaneous physical metamorphosis. Many of us would like the process of evolution to stop after puberty. The *I Ching*, one of the cornerstones of Chinese philosophy, tells us that all the suffering of mankind is produced by attachment to a previous condition of existence. We try to hold on to what we were up until yesterday. We cannot bring back last Tuesday. If we continue thinking as we did last summer, while the entire galaxy and the whole universe has shifted its configuration, our thought pattern vibrates disharmonically with the basic energy pattern of the cosmos. The body translates this disharmony into physical symptoms.

Freud and Piaget, among others, have emphasized that the very young child does not differentiate between ego and environment. It is aware of events, but not of itself as a separate entity. It lives in a state of mental symbiosis in the womb. The universe is focussed on the self, and the self *is* the universe—a condition which Piaget called 'protoplasmic' or 'symbiotic' consciousness, and which may be at the origin of that 'oceanic feeling' which the artist and the mystic strive to recapture on a high level of development, at a higher turn of the spiral. Symbiotic consciousness is never completely defeated, merely relegated underground to those primitive strata in the mental hierarchy where the boundaries of the ego are still fluid and blurred. It survives in the sympathetic magic of primitives, the belief in transubstantiation, the mystic bonds which unite a person with his tribe, his totem, his shadow, his effigy, and later with his god. In the major Eastern philosophies, the 'I am thou and thou are me,' the identity of the 'real self' with the Atman, the all-one, has been preserved throughout the ages.

All non-Cartesian cosmologies postulate the existence of a vibratory essence which permeates and creates our symbiotic conscious experience, and call it by a variety of names—God, Chi (Qi), prana, bioplasma, etc. In Chinese medical philosophy, Chi is a flow of blood and lymph and nervous impulses,...which follows well-defined pathways called meridians. According to the Chinese explanation, whenever the flow of this energy along the meridians is either obstructed or weakened, the likelihood for sickness is increased. This functional disturbance of energy flow can produce the organic and structural changes associated with disease.

It is proposed that we all exist suspended in a sea of energy which penetrates between and through our body cells. The neutrino, an uncharged elementary particle that is believed to be massless, is an energy form known to possess this capability. Arthur Koestler describes it (in his *Roots of Coincidence*) as having "virtually no mass, no electric charge, no magnetic field. It is not attracted by gravity, nor captured or repelled by the electric and magnetic fields of other particles while flying past them. Accordingly, a neutrino originating in the Milky Way, or even in some other galaxy, and travelling with the speed of light, can go clean through the solid body of the earth as if it were so much empty space... A neutrino can be stopped only by a direct, head-on collision with another elementary particle, and the chances of such a direct collision ... are estimated at about one in ten thousand million... The absence of 'gross' physical properties in the neutrino and its quasi-ethereal character, encouraged speculations about the possible existence of other particles which would provide the missing link between matter and mind."

Our physical body is conceived to be widely separated islands of particulate matter suspended in this energy soup which also makes thought. The sum total of this energy is called Chi (Qi). In traditional Chinese medicine Chi is said to fall into two main categories: the force of daytime energy, or light, is called *yang*; the night force, the energy of darkness, is called *yin*. Chi is the resultant or combination of these complementary equipotent forces. In the summer the light, yang aspect of Chi is predominant, while in the winter the night, yin facet of cosmic energy overpowers the light. The days grow shorter, the nights longer, until the winter solstice. The light power, on the brink of extinction, changes its direction and begins to grow stronger at the expense of its eternal opponent. This polarity reversal is depicted in all the pagan myths of the sun god who dies and is resurrected. It occurs because anything pushed to its extreme turns into the opposite according to the Tao, the creative principle that orders the universe. In the Western world we refer to the energy as God or cosmic energy. Our entire organism, every cell in the body, pulsates harmonically with the light/dark alternations which create a day. The balance between rest and activity parallels exactly the seasonal yin/yang, dark/light, relationship. In 24 hours, one earth revolution, Chi energy makes a complete circuit of the body and reenters the cosmic sea. This accounts for the phenomenon of *circadian* (approximately daily) rhythms, cyclic variations in biologic activity in all living systems: cells, organisms, and even groups of organisms, the tides of life.

The reply to the Yellow Emperor by his physician, circa 3000 B.C., sheds some light on the reasons why Cro-Magnon displays tendencies toward greater longevity in his primitive state than he does in his civilized state: "In ancient times, people patterned themselves on the principles of nature and lived in harmony (with the seasons). Nowadays, people are not like this... Their passions exhaust their vital forces; their cravings dissipate their true essence. They do not know how to find contentment within themselves; they are not skilled in the control of their spirits; they devote all their attention to the amusement of their minds, cutting themselves off from the joys of long life. Their rising and retiring is without regularity. For these reasons they reach only one half the hundred years and then they degenerate."

There's another way of looking at it. Einstein's admonition warns that our concepts regarding external reality are not identical with that reality. A case in point is the dispute between Galileo and the Catholic heirarchy over the cause of the apparent motion of the sun across the sky. The church, supported by the common sense evidence available to the eyes of anyone who took the trouble to look, forced him under threat of torture to recant his idea that the earth was actually moving in space; not only that, but rotating too! When he admitted that the sun was really moving around the stationary earth as it seemed to be doing, a noted author of that period wrote: "The disputes of Signor Galileo have dissolved into alchemical smoke. so here we are at last, safely back on solid earth, and we do not have to fly with it as so many ants on a balloon." Einstein's theory of relativity settled the argument with the observation that "absolute motion is impossible to determine." Dr. Joseph Cambpell tells us that: "the world itself, it is said by some, is...an ink blot in which different people see different forms, symptomatic of the psychology of their own fantasizing minds."

Both agree that things are rarely what they seem. Observation of any phenomenon is a factor which affects the thing being observed. In the light of this and other considerations, we may safely assume along with Jung, Plato, and Schopenhauer that absolute reality like absolute motion, is impossible to determine. he alchemists view of reality 'tam ethice quam physice' (as psychical as it is physical) is another way of seeing the world as an ink blot. The Buddhist version is an image of the moon on the water whose clarity depends on the state of calm of the water's surface (the mind of the observer). Modern scientific method calms the waters by requiring detached observation of empirical data. 19th and early 20th century science differed sharply with alchemical theory when it split into a pair of opposites: the scientist's observing psyche vs. the natural phenomenon under observation. Alchemists like the mathematician Pythagoras, and Paracelus, the physician (who founded the science of modern chemotherapeutics) maintained that the two, the ink blot, and the psyche which is examining that ink blot, were complementary aspects of a single indivisible reality. Wolfgang Pauli, a quantum physicist who worked closely with Carl Jung describes modern science's tilt toward alchemy:

> The general problem of the relationship between mind and body, between the inward and the outward, cannot be said to have been solved by the concept of psychophysical parallelism postulated in the last century. Modern science has perhaps brought us nearer to a more satisfactory understanding of this relationship, by introducing the concept of complementarity into physics itself. It would be the more satisfactory solution if mind and body could be interpreted as complementary aspects of the same reality.

This statement has enormous implications for those of us who would be physicians and healers, if we are not to dismiss the most respected scientists of our time as "closet alchemists." It sheds a great deal of light on the current controversy about acupuncture therapeutics.

As recently as 1970, the conventional wisdom of Western medical orthodoxy dismissed acupuncture as pure quackery. The acupuncture system, it was claimed, existed only in the minds of the quaint yellow practitioners of the cult, and the cures, if any, existed only in the minds of the deluded patients. The accepted technical term for this kind of cure was, and still is, "the placebo effect." Dr. Jesse Wexler, a young physician who worked at the Headlands Clinic for two years instead of serving the ends of the Vietnam War, referred to those who held the orthodox view as "cement heads." When reports of acupuncture-induced cures began coming in from China, Germany, France and the USSR, the cement heads began to give ground. Having seen with their own eyes the removal of lungs and thyroid glands (at Shanghai General Hospital) under acupuncture anethesia, they admitted the obvious. Acupuncture anesthesia seemed as effective as the infinitely more expensive brand practiced in our infinitely superior Western hospitals. Its success in altering the course of physical disease was ascribed to hypnosis, somehow related to the well-known brainwashing techniques practices by godless communism. The anesthetic effect remained, and demanded an explanation which would preserve the cement head cosmology. The explanation, taken from the advertising copy for a machine called the 'A-Alpha Activator for Electronic Analgesia' is as follows:

"The A-Alpha Activator is a device designed for the suppression of chronic pain. It is based on the gate theory of pain inhibition first promulgated by Wall and Associates which, briefly summarized, states that the sensation of pain is conducted at a much slower rate than normal sensations of touch, pressure, vibration, and so forth. Normal sensations are carried along fibers known as A-Alpha fibers and, according to the gate theory, when these fibers are stimulated they will close a hypothetical 'gate' in the spinal cord which then inhibits the conduction of pain impulses."

In his *Roots of Coincidence*, Arthur Koestler notes the observation of Sir John Eddington that "the stuff of the world is mind stuff." He concludes that "the hard, tangible appearance of things exist only in our medium-sized world measured in pounds and yards, to which our senses are attuned. On both the cosmic and the subatomic scale this intimate, tangible relationship turns out to be an illusion." The gate which inhibits pain is a figment of the imagination of P. D. Wall as much as the acupuncture system is a figment of the imagination of the Yellow Emperor's chief physician. At best it is 'a physical concept which however it may seem, is not exclusively determined by external reality.'

A well-known neurophysiologist, Norman Shealy, M.D., invented a device known as the "dorsal column stimulator" which, by closing the hallucinatory gate of P. D. Wall and associates, relieves severe, intractible pain caused by a variety of pathologic conditions. Newer adaptations of this technique require only that a small electric current be applied to the skin over the areas along the spine. It is no longer necessary to implant the electrodes directly into the spinal cord. Arthur Winter, M.D., who has used the transcutaneous (across the skin) method reports "patients suffering from acute pain involving the neck, back and lower spine due to various causes, such as arthritis and cancer were relieved with transcutaneous nerve stimulation where other methods failed." By naming his procedure as he does, Dr. Winter implies a mode of action for his pain relieving procedure. Transcutaneous nerve stimulation, like the gate theory remains an unproven physical concept or theory. We only know that a small electric current applied to the back relieves intractible pain. The exact nature of pain and its detailed method of transmission are, according to the beginning of Dr. Winter's report, unknown. He brings to mind Wolfgang Pauli's concept of psychosomatic unity and identity when he states that "the gate control theory of Wall and Melzack...does not take into account the higher levels of influence from descending impulses from the brain." Dr. Lowenschuss of Columbia University thinks that small electric currents applied to the skin invariably seek out the acupuncture points which show decreased resistance to the flow of electricity. If we buy this view, then we must consider transcutaneous nerve stimulation to be a form of electroacupuncture. The New Jersey State Legislature is considering a bill which declares that acupuncture is really a form of physiotherapy. Where is the truth in this controversy? Which point of view, we may ask, is the closest to objective reality?

Professor Einstein offers us a guideline:

"The simpler our picture of the external world, and the more facts it embraces, the stronger it reflects in our mind the harmony of the universe."

As we enter the last quarter of the 20th century, the alchemical picture of the world has achieved wide recognition and acceptance among our most gifted scientific minds. In his *Roots of Coincidence*, Arthur Koestler quotes one such, Sir James Jeans, as follows:

"Today there is a wide measure of agreement, which on the physical side of science approaches almost to unanimity, that the stream of knowledge is heading toward a non-mechanical reality; the universe begins to look more like a great thought than a great machine." (The date was 1937!)

Tam ethice quam physice!

The theme was taken up in an article which appeared in *Medical World News* in the early 70s of the dying 20th century. It bore the title, "Scanning Electron Microscopy." The problem is that scientists cannot now understand the structures they visualize at magnifications of tens of thousands of diameters. The living world, which we have been examining through the 440 power eyes of the optical medical microscope is unrecognizable. Compare the view of the forest floor of an elephant to that of an ant! The single cell, which to the 440 power elephant is the simplest constituent of living tissue has, in the elephantine view a nucleus, some cytoplasm, an apparatus for division, and some other bodies which he leaves to the chemists to investigate. The electronic ant on the other hand, sees an intricately complex factory whose structure we have not even begun to understand. The electron microscopist sees in a drop of blood the primeval sea; a saline solution inhabited by living creatures whose shapes and appearances compare with the wildest flights of the imagination, stoned or sober. It has been suggested by some, according to the *Medical World News* article, that we must now completely revise our early concepts of pathology and physiology of living tissue.

The elephant's eye view has led to physical concepts which may be considered outmoded for several reasons, not the least of which is its dismal failure in the field of healing and the alleviation of human suffering. The cell, we now know, when magnified a million times is a structure as complex as the gross organism from which it comes. The microscopist, the physicist and the astronomers who are trying to understand the significance of things like black holes in space have all come up against the same ink blot. The huge Rorschach that we call empirical reality seems to be infinitely large, and similarly and equally complex at the big and the small ends. The statement, "as above so below," succinctly summarizes the modern scientific picture of the ink blot. It is attributed to Hermes Trismegistus, an ancient figure said to have been a physician, who is closely associated with the symbol of 20th century medicine, the caduceus.

Our new medical model must be built on a firm foundation. The theories of Einstein, de Chardin and Jung seem like sturdy supporting pillars. In Einstein's cosmos, says Koestler, matter dissolves into energy, energy into shifting configurations of something unknown. Is this something the mind which Dr. Pauli considers to be a complementary aspect of the body? Dr. Jung and other modern psychiatrists call it the psyche. The human body is as much an energy packet consisting of wave phenomena as it is solid lump of accumulated particles obeying only the laws of Newtonian physics. We may postulate that a beam of high frequency sound, like a beam of congruent light from a laser, irons out standing waves in the acupuncture meridian system. Standing waves, in which energy is stagnant, precipitate the matter of the physical body as deformed or diseased tissues.

Pain relief and restoration of normal bodily function have been the 'raison d'etre' (the justification) for the existence of the healing profession since the dawn of recorded history. The degree to which we can achieve these objectives is the yardstick or standard of performance against which humanity has always measured the work of its physicians. It is still so. The work of Shealy, Winter and others in the area of pain relief indicate that pain, about whose nature and mode of transmission we know nothing, can be controlled by the application of a non-specific stimulus (electricity) to a part of the body apparently unrelated to the part that hurts. Dr. Shealy's dorsal column stimulator shoots a small electrical stimulus directly into the spinal column somewhere between the source of the pain and the brain. It has been shown to be effective in pain in the lower part of the back and the legs where all else had failed. (This therapeutic approach was rejected as an alternative for our patients because it requires a dangerous and expensive surgical operation.) The A-Alpha activator and Winters' transcutaneous nerve stimulator seemed simpler and far safer procedures, and there was convincing clinical evidence that they worked. Columbia University's Dr. Lowenschuss' suggestion that small electric currents stimulate not nerve trunks, but acupuncture points is a valid contention. If he is right, then any other form of vibratory energy could provide the necessary stimulus (if applied directly to these electrical windows in the living skin), to duplicate the results of Shealy and Winters. The acupuncture points are the black holes in space of 20th century medical research. Stimulating them with vibratory energy seems to stop chronic, severe, and intractible pain due to a variety of causes.

It is also possible to convert the physical symptom into a mind picture. The patient concentrates on his pain or problem and waits for a visual image to appear spontaneously. This image often takes the form which Jung describes as a 'mandala.' The term 'mandala' was chosen because this word denotes the ritual or magic circle used in Lamaism and also in Tantric yoga as an aid to contemplation. The spontaneous appearance of a mandala symbol is accompanied by healing on the physical plane according to Dr. Jung. Further elucidation of these concepts with examples of commonly experienced mandalas can be found in *Psychology and Alchemy* and Jung's smaller work entitled *Mandala Symbolism*.

Teilhard de Chardin, the Jesuit-paleontologist, in his *Phenomenon of Man*, agrees that consciousness and matter are two faces of a single metaprocess. Inherent in the nature of this metaprocess is the tendency to evolve, by simultaneously amplifying its conscious aspect and 'complexifying' its matter aspect. Hydrogen ions, he feels, are as much a spark of consciousness as a speck of matter. (Here again we meet the alchemical 'tam ethice, quam physice' and the Einsteinian wave particle or wavicle.) The evolution of the metaprocess from hydrogen atom to conscious human is discontinuous. It takes place in a series of steps or quantum leaps. One such leap was the introduction of life on the planet. Another took place when the first specimen of that life became conscious.

Jung refers to this primal urge to evolve when he says: "There is within the psyche a process that seeks its own goal independently of external factors." His technique of healing through the modality of 'active imagination' is simple:

"Choose a dream, or some other fantasy image and concentrate on it by simply looking at it. You can also use a bad mood (or physical symptom) as a starting point. Try to find out what image expresses this mood (or symptom). Fix this image in your mind by concentrating on it. Usually it will alter, as the mere fact of contemplating it animates it."

In our own version of the 'mystical marriage' between conscious and unconscious, we suggest to our patients that they will see figures of either sex whom they are to consider to be the representatives of their unconscious psyche (the rest of the universe). Jung's description continued: "In this way conscious and unconscious are united."

At first there is a tendency to watch these figures much as one would watch a television movie. In other words, you dream with open eyes. This description coincides with a process developed at the Menninger Clinic by the Drs. Green known as 'Theta Reverie' (*vide supra*). "The piece that is being played does not want merely to be watched, it wants to compel participation. The observer will notice, as the actors appear, one by one, and the plot thickens that they all have some purposeful relationship to his conscious situation, that he is being addressed by the unconscious, and that *it* causes these fantasy figures to appear before him."

The fantasy figures, if accepted by the patient as real, in the Jungian sense, will enter into dialogue with him (her). If asked, "Did you cause my illness?" the figures often respond affirmatively. If asked, "What are you trying to tell me?" or "Why are you mad at me?" the imaginary helper or guide responds with information which is exquisitely relevant to the deepest layers of the questioner's psychic and physical being.

Noting that what he calls "coming to terms with the unconscious," the alchemists called "meditation," Jung quotes the following alchemical definition:

"Meditation: the name of an internal talk of one person with another who is invisible, as in the invocation of the Diety, or communion with one's self, or with one's good angel." The goal of this meditation is the creation of wholeness; a condition of hoemostasis or balance between two opposite and complementary aspects of every human being. The crowned hermaphrodite on Barry's 'Jung tee shirt' symbolized this state of consciousness which is that of a single being simultaneously male and female, conscious and unconscious.

Compare Heisenberg's concept of complementarity as

known to modern physics, which states that only the juxaposi-tion of two mutually exclusive and contradictory frames of reference (i.e. male and female) provide an exhaustive view of the appearances of phenomena (empirical reality).

The *conversation* is a manifestation of energy flow between the two hemispheres. This takes place through two connecting nerve bundles called the *Corpus Callosum* and the *anterior commissure*. The appearance of the apparition indi-cates flow of energy from female to male hemispheres. Energy flowing between the hemispheres tends to rebalance itself. The resultant flow down the spinal cord via the hypothalmus tends to correct pathogenic imbalance manifesting somatic disease. This happens only if the *ego* follows the advice of the *helper*.

The phenomenon *man* manifests (as does every other con-ceivable phenomenon) in two aspects. *Ego*, who manifests *my liver*, and the *Helper*, or *Cro-Magnon*, who grows *the liver*. Ego-Man at any point in his life is faced with a pressure from his Cro-Magnon unconscious. He is constrained to continue the process of human evolution. Continuous conscious growth is the price of survival. Each quantum growth step is a birth. Each birth is in essence a death. Evolution seems to be the entity which creates the opposites of birth and death. It is at these critical periods of change that it is essential for us to remain quiet and receptive.

If we, like King Canute who ordered the tide to stop coming in, set our will against the tide of evolution, our mental vibratory rate becomes disharmonic with the basic pre-vailing field of mind pattern. We become a maladapted organism in a rapidly changing environment. The result, as in the case of the dinosaur, is inevitable. Our small, ego-centered experience is the vehicle for human evolution. It is in each one of us that mankind lives and expresses itself. The mysterious process which initiates and directs our embryonic develop-ment, that which grows us arms and legs, does not end at birth. It persists all of our lives, changing our ego state constantly and irrevocably, fetus to child, to adult, to oldster. *We only have to know that the process means us no harm.* Attachment to any previous state is equivalent to the refusal of a fetus to be born. The ego's attempt to oppose the forces of nature invites physical destruction.

If humanity is indeed evolving it is conceivable that the play of cosmic energy sets the pattern and the direction for the evolutionary process. If an individual encloses himself in an ego-centered little box, the chances are that he or she will be recycled. A human who refuses to evolve is like a fetus which refuses to be born. These evolutionary changes happen in steps or quantum jumps. The birth process is the prototype. When cosmic or bioplasmic energy changes its configuration, we must adapt and agree to be someone else. to evolve means to die to all that went before, and to be born into a strange new body, mind, and life situation. The egress from the womb is a one-way, irrevocable transition as is the change of puberty. Just as it is impossible to reverse the birth process, it is also impossible to resist it. As Bob Dylan says, "Whoever is not busy being born is busy dyin'."

Medical practitioners must place themselves within this evolutionary framework. Cures are being noted in unrelated diseases by procedures which fly in the face of Cartesian rationalism. Since the evidence is undeniable, current theory must be modified. The prime function of the general practitioner is that of making his patients feel better. *Any procedure which offers relief of human suffering must be investigated.* Theoretical objections to the rationality of the method must take second place, or be left to the theoreticians. 20th century medicine has failed to provide satisfactory resolution to the vast majority of our health problems. This is because it is based on a 16th century paradigm. As the 21st century approaches, we must be willing to discard discredited and obsolete assumptions. Man's world picture continues to evolve independently of his consciousness and will.

The process of looking within for advice and guidance is the foundation stone for the therapeutic approach of Carl Jung and of the other alchemists. He maintains that if life is not going well, it is to be considered that the self, consisting of the totality of consciousness plus the entire realm of unconscious life processes, holds the key. All the energy in the universe which is not our own consciousness can communicate with us. The imaginary figure our patients make up seems to be a means by which each one of us can get in touch with his or her own self.

The alchemical process is summarized in the axiomatic *solve et coagula;* it involves a separation and a subsequent reunion. There must be a separation from, and a withdrawal of, identification with the ego state. This is accomplished by meditation which puts the thinker into alpha and silences him like switching a radio from AM to FM. Just as you can't get an FM station on an AM radio, it is not possible to pay attention to thoughts and the process of active imagination simultaneously.

The search for the panacea, healing energy, begins with a raw material which is so cheap and plentiful that people do not even look at it—a contemptible fantasy. Accept the fact that our unconscious can give us valuable insights and meditate or observe your own imagery for 15–20 minutes daily. Drawing the images helps make them clearer and more definite. It is possible to think of the images as holographic pictures which represent the changing patterns of the universal energy flux. These pictures give one a cosmic weather report which, like terrestrial weather reports, help us navigate our course through daily life.

At this point in our research, we suggest that visual imagery techniques be used in addition to standard medical techniques. It is well to consider the method of visual imagery as something to do until the doctor comes, or perhaps something to do if he has pronounced: "There is nothing more that can be done!"

FOOTNOTES

1. A preliminary report on this group was published as "Acupuncture with High Frequency Sound," in *OP/The Osteopathic Physician*, September 1973.
2. Meyer Friedman & Ray H. Roseman, *Type A Behavior and Your Heart*. New York: Knopf, 1974.
3. Hans Selye, *Stress of Life*. New York: McGraw-Hill, 1956.
4. Hans Selye, "The Evolution of the Stress Concept," *American Scientist*, November-December, 1973.
5. William H. Glazier, "The Task of Medicine," *Scientific American*, March 1973.
6. World Health Organization.
7. "Drug Firms Back Big Promotions," *Washington Post*, March 13, 1974.
8. *Annals of Internal Medicine*, October 1973.
9. Elmer E. Green, Alyce M. Green, and E. Dale Walters, "Voluntary Control of Internal States: Psychological and Physiological," *Transpersonal Psychology*, Vol. II, No. 1, 1970.
10. Jack Leahy, "Controlling the Mind," *OP/The Osteopathic Physician*, June 1974.
11. Carl Simonton, M.D., "The Role of the Mind in Cancer Therapy," *The Dimensions of Healing*. Los Altos, CA.: The Academy of Parapsychology and Medicine, 1972.
12. Bertrand Russell, *An Outline of Philosophy*. New York: World Publishing Co. Originally published in 1927.
13. Alan Watts, *The Essence of Alan Watts: Nothingness*. Millbrae, CA.: Celestial Arts, 1974.
14. Dr. Jeffery J. Smith, "The Occult and the Intellectual." *Parapsychology Review*, May-June 1974.
15. "Finger-Tip Halos of Kirlian Photography," *Medical World News*, October 26, 1973.
16. H. S. Dakin, *High-Voltage Photography*. San Francisco: Dakin, 1974.
17. Douglas Dean, "High Voltage Phototherapy Applied to Psychic Healing," *Dimensions of Healing*. Los Altos, CA.: The Academy of Parapsychology and Medicine, 1972.

BIBLIOGRAPHY

Acupuncture Anaesthesia. Peking: Foreign Languages Press, 1972

Bedrij, Orest *Yes It's Love: Your Life Can Be A Miracle.* New York: Family Library, 1974.

Birns, H.D. *Hypnosis.* New York: Award Books, 1968.

Caprio, Frank S., M.D. and Joseph R. Berger *Helping Yourself with Self-Hypnosis.* Englewood Cliffs, N.J.: Prentice-Hall, 1963.

Cerney, J.V. *Acupuncture Without Needles.* West Nyack, N.Y.: Parker Publishing Company, 1974.

Chen, Ronald *The History and Methods of Physical Diagnosis in Classical Chinese Medicine.* New York: Vantage Press, 1969.

Clark, Adrian V. *Psycho-Kinesis: Moving Matter with the Mind.* West Nyack, N.Y.: Parker Publishing Company, 1973.

Clark, Linda, *Help Yourself to Health.* New York: Pyramid Books, 1974.

Duke, Marc *Acupuncture.* New York: Pyramid Books, 1973.

Ebon, Martin (editor) *Psychic Discoveries by the Russians.* New York: New American Library, 1971.

Edwards, E.D. (editor) *The Dragon Book.* London: William Hodge and Co., Ltd., 1946.

Edwards, Harry *The Healing Intelligence.* New York: Taplinger Publishing Company, 1971.

Exploring the Secrets of Treating Deaf-Mutes. Peking: Foreign Language Press, 1972.

Gross, Don *The Case for Spiritual Healing.* New York: Thomas Nelson & Sons, 1958.

Hammond, Sally *We Are All Healers.* New York: Harper & Row, 1973.

Hartley-Hennessy, T. *Healing by Water or Drinking Sunlight and Oxygen.* Durban, South Africa: Essence of Health Publishing Co., 1966.

Hashimoto, Masae *Japanese Acupuncture.* London: Thorsons Publishers, 1966.

Holzer, Hans *Beyond Medicine.* Chicago: Henry Regnery Company, 1973.

Huard, Pierre and Ming Wong *Chinese Medicine.* New York: McGraw-Hill, 1968.

Hume, Edward Hicks *The Chinese Way in Medicine.* Baltimore: The Johns Hopkins University Press, 1940.

Iklin, A. Graham *New Concepts of Healing*. London: Hodder and Stoughton, 1955.

Jones, D.C. *Spiritual Healing*. New York: Longmans, Green & Co., 1955.

Jones, E. Stanley *Abundant Living*. Nashville, Tenn.: Abingdon Press, 1942.

Kreig, Margaret B. *Green Medicine: The Search for Plants that Heal*. Chicago: Rand McNally & Company, 1964.

Lavier, Dr. J. (translation by Dr. Philip M. Chancellor) *Points of Chinese Acupuncture*. Rustington, Sussex, England: Health Science Press, 1965.

Lawrence, Jodi *Alpha Brain Waves*. Los Angeles: Nash Publishing Corporation, 1972.

Lawson-Wood, Denis and Joyce Lawson-Wood *Five Elements of Acupuncture and Chinese Massage*. Rustington, England: Health Science Press, 1965.

Lawson-Wood, Denis and Joyce Lawson-Wood *Judo: Revival Points, Athletes' Points, and Posture*. Rustington, England: Health Science Press, 1960.

LeShan, Lawrence *The Medium, the Mystic, and the Physicist*. New York: The Viking Press, 1974.

Loewe, Michael *Everyday Life in Early Imperial China*. New York: G.P. Putnam's Sons, 1968.

Longgood William *The Poisons in Your Food*. New York: Simon and Schuster, 1960.

Mann, Felix *The Meridians of Acupuncture*. London: William Heinemann Medical Books, 1964.

Marriott, Alice and Carol K. Rachlin *Peyote*. New York: Thomas Y. Crowell Company, 1971.

Martin, Bernard *Healing for You*. Richmond, Va.: John Knox Press, 1965.

Maxwell, Nicole *Witch Doctor's Apprentice*. Boston: Houghton Mifflin Company, 1961.

Meyer, Clarence *American Folk Medicine*. New York: Thomas Y. Crowell Company, 1973.

Montgomery, D. Wayne (editor) *Healing and Wholeness*. Richmond, Va.: John Knox Press, 1971.

Naranjo, Claudio *The Healing Journey: New Approaches to Consciousness*. New York: Pantheon Books, 1973.

Neal, Emily Gardiner *God Can Heal You Now*. Englewood Cliffs, N.J.: Prentice-Hall, 1958.

Nittler, Alan H., M.D. *A New Breed of Doctor*. New York: Pyramid House, 1972.

Ostrander, Sheila and Lynn Schroeder *Psychic Discoveries Behind the Iron Curtain.* Englewood Cliffs, N.J.: Prentice-Hall, 1970.

Oursler, Will *The Healing Power of Faith.* New York: Hawthorn Books, 1957.

Parkhurst, Genevieve *Healing the Whole Person.* New York, N.Y.: Morehouse-Barlow Co., 1968.

Puharich, Andrija *Uri: A Journal of the Mystery of Uri Geller.* Garden City, N.Y.: Anchor Press, 1974.

Sniveley, William Daniel, Jr., M.D. and Jan Theurbach *Healing Beyond Medicine.* West Nyack, N.Y.: Parker Publishing Company, 1972.

Tester, M.H. *The Healing Touch.* New York: Taplinger Publishing Company, 1970.

Veith, Ilza *The Yellow Emperor's Classic of Internal Medicine.* Berkeley, California: University of California Press, 1966.

Vithoulkas, George *Homeopathy: Medicine of the New Man.* New York: Avon Books, 1972.

Waerland, Ebba *Rebuilding Health.* Old Greenwich, Conn.: The Devin-Adair Co., 1961.

Warmbrand, Max, N.D., D.O. *The Encyclopedia of Natural Health.* New York: The Julian Press, 1962.

Wing Tsit-chan (editor) *A Source Book in Chinese Philosophy.* Princeton: The Princeton University Press, 1950.

Woodard, Christopher *A Doctor Heals by Faith.* London: Max Parrish Co., Ltd., 1953.

Zaffuto, Anthony A., Ph.D., with Mary Q. Zaffuto *Alphagenics: How to Use Your Brain Waves to Improve Your Life.* Garden City, N.Y.: Doubleday & Company, Inc., 1974.

INDEX

BIOGRAPHY

DR. IRVING OYLE OF BOLINAS

What makes a 49-year-old osteopath from New York move to a California coastal town and give up a lucrative general practice for "healing"?

Since graduating from the Philadelphia College of Osteopathic Medicine in 1953, Dr. Oyle has been undergoing an evolution. After interning at Mercy Douglas and Metropolitan Hospitals in Philadelphia, he entered private general practice in Farmingdale, New York.

In 1966 he volunteered to run a hospital and health clinic in Mexico operated for the Tarahumara Indians. His brief stay that summer convinced him that there was more to healing than could be found in modern textbooks and hospitals. He sold the lucrative practice in Farmingdale and opened a storefront clinic on the lower east side of Manhattan.

Finally, after two years in the clinic and another trip to Mexico, Dr. Oyle decided to move his investigations to an area more conducive to research. (He chose Bolinas because of his love for the ocean.) He found the Presbyterian Synod of the Golden Gate was willing to take an active role in establishing a clinic in the town of Bolinas and he was able to begin "to investigate just what it is that causes healing."

During the first years of the Headlands Healing Service, Dr. Oyle wrote a book *Magic, Mysticism and Modern Medicine*, telling of his experiences and revealing the controversial direction of his healing practices.

Now in the "middle of the experiment," he is not willing to claim drastic departure from the bounds of orthodox Western medicine: "Don't put me in the spook section, I'm just a family doctor turned medical researcher, trying to find out what it is that gets people well. And approaching the job with an open mind."

As of *The Healing Mind*, Dr. Oyle is open enough to include acupuncture-sonopuncture, mind control, biofeedback, mental imagery, yoga, Jungian psychology, and alchemy to cause healing. But, because he is "growing" hourly, he has already moved into other realms since writing this book.

CELESTIAL ARTS BOOK LIST

LOVE IS AN ATTITUDE, poetry and photographs by Walter Rinder.
03-0 Paper @ $3.95   04-9 Cloth @ $7.95

THIS TIME CALLED LIFE, poetry and photographs by Walter Rinder.
05-7 Paper @ $3.95   06-5 Cloth @ $7.95

SPECTRUM OF LOVE, poetry by Walter Rinder with David Mitchell art.
19-7 Paper @ $2.95   20-0 Cloth @ $7.95

FOLLOW YOUR HEART, poetry by Walter Rinder with Richard Davis art.
39-1 Paper @ $2.95

THE HUMANNESS OF YOU, Vol. 1, art and philosophy by Walter Rinder.
47-2 Paper @ $2.95

THE HUMANNESS OF YOU, Vol. 2, art and philosophy by Walter Rinder.
54-5 Paper @ $2.95

VISIONS OF YOU, poetry by George Betts and photography by Robert Scales.
07-3 Paper @ $3.95

MY GIFT TO YOU, poetry by George Betts and photography by Robert Scales.
15-4 Paper @ $3.95

YOU & I, poetry and photography by Leonard Nimoy.
26-X Paper @ $3.95   27-8 Cloth @ $7.95

WILL I THINK OF YOU?, poetry and photography by Leonard Nimoy.
70-7 Paper @ $3.95

SPEAK THEN OF LOVE, poetry by Andrew Oerke with Asian art.
29-4 Paper @ $3.95

I AM, concepts of awareness in poetic form by Michael Grinder with color art.
25-1 Paper @ $2.95

GAMES STUDENTS PLAY, transactional analysis in schools by Ken Ernst.
16-2 Paper @ $3.95   17-0 Cloth @ $7.95

GUIDE FOR SINGLE PARENTS, transactional analysis by Kathryn Hallett.
55-3 Paper @ $3.95   64-2 Cloth @ $7.95

PASSIONATE MIND, guidance and understanding by Joel Kramer.
63-4 Paper @ $3.95

SENSIBLE BOOK, understanding children's senses by Barbara Polland.
53-7 Paper @ $3.95

THIS TIMELESS MOMENT, Aldous Huxley's life by Laura Huxley.
22-5 Paper @ $4.95

HOW TO BE SOMEBODY, a guide for personal growth by Yetta Bernhard.
20-9 Paper @ $4.95

CREATIVE SURVIVAL, the problems of single mothers by Persia Woolley.
17-9 Paper @ $4.95

FAT LIBERATION, the awareness technique to losing weight by Alan Dolit.
03-9 Paper @ $3.95

ALPHA BRAIN WAVES, explanation of same by D. Boxerman and A. Spilken.
16-0 Paper @ $4.95

INWARD JOURNEY, art as therapy by Margaret Keyes.
81-2 Paper @ $4.95

GOD, poetic visions of the abstract by Alan Watts.
75-8 Paper @ $3.95

Write for a free catalog to:
CELESTIAL ARTS   231 Adrian Road   Millbrae, California 94030